SEX AND SEXUALITY IN MEDIEVAL ENGLAND

SEX AND SEXUALITY IN MEDIEVAL ENGLAND

KATHRYN WARNER

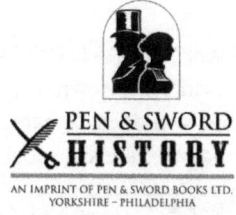

PEN & SWORD HISTORY

AN IMPRINT OF PEN & SWORD BOOKS LTD.
YORKSHIRE – PHILADELPHIA

First published in Great Britain in 2022 by
PEN AND SWORD HISTORY
An imprint of
Pen & Sword Books Ltd
Yorkshire – Philadelphia

Copyright © Kathryn Warner, 2022

ISBN 978 1 39909 832 8

The right of Kathryn Warner to be identified as Author of
this work has been asserted by her in accordance with the Copyright,
Designs and Patents Act 1988.

A CIP catalogue record for this book is available from the British Library.

All rights reserved. No part of this book may be reproduced or transmitted in
any form or by any means, electronic or mechanical including photocopying,
recording or by any information storage and retrieval system, without permission
from the Publisher in writing.

Typeset in Times New Roman 11.5/14 by
SJmagic DESIGN SERVICES, India.
Printed and bound in the UK by CPI Group (UK) Ltd.

Pen & Sword Books Limited incorporates the imprints of Atlas, Archaeology,
Aviation, Discovery, Family History, Fiction, History, Maritime, Military, Military
Classics, Politics, Select, Transport, True Crime, Air World, Frontline Publishing,
Leo Cooper, Remember When, Seaforth Publishing, The Praetorian Press,
Wharncliffe Local History, Wharncliffe Transport, Wharncliffe True Crime and
White Owl.

For a complete list of Pen & Sword titles please contact
PEN & SWORD BOOKS LIMITED
47 Church Street, Barnsley, South Yorkshire, S70 2AS, England
E-mail: enquiries@pen-and-sword.co.uk
Website: www.pen-and-sword.co.uk

Or
PEN AND SWORD BOOKS
1950 Lawrence Rd, Havertown, PA 19083, USA
E-mail: Uspen-and-sword@casematepublishers.com
Website: www.penandswordbooks.com

Contents

Kings of England in the Later Middle Ages viii
Money ix
Introduction x

Chapter 1   Appearance 1
             Cleanliness 1
             Clothing 4

Chapter 2   Marriage (1) 9
             Age at Marriage 9
             Weddings 15
             Wedding Customs 17
             Present and Future Vows 19

Chapter 3   Marriage (2) 21
             Clandestine Marriages and Bigamy 21
             Marriage Rights 23
             Rank 28

Chapter 4   Marriage (3) 32
             Second Marriages 32
             Dowry 35
             Dower and the Courtesy of England 36

Chapter 5   Marriage (4) 38
             Abductions and Forced Marriages 38
             Disputed and Unhappy Marriages 42
             Impediments and Domestic Abuse 45

Chapter 6	Sexual Pleasure and Relationships (1)	49
	Sexual Pleasure and Desire	49
	Virginity and Chastity	51
Chapter 7	Sexual Pleasure and Relationships (2)	55
	Adultery and Pre-Marital Sex	55
	Unchaste Ecclesiastics	61
Chapter 8	Love Language	64
Chapter 9	Pregnancy and Childbirth (1)	68
	Menstruation	68
	Conception and Contraception	68
	Miscarriages and Abortions	70
Chapter 10	Pregnancy and Childbirth (2)	73
	Examining Women's Bodies	73
	Birth Aids and Customs	74
	Midwives	77
	Multiple Births	78
	Mortality Rates in Childbirth and Infancy	80
Chapter 11	Pregnancy and Childbirth (3)	83
	Baptism and Godparents	83
	Purification	87
	Wet-Nurses	88
	Family Size	90
	Parents' Ages	92
Chapter 12	Illegitimacy	95
Chapter 13	Prostitution	103
Chapter 14	Ravishment and Abduction	108
	Age of Consent	108
	Ravishment/Rape	110
	Child Abuse	115

Contents

Chapter 15   Incest and Consanguinity 117

Chapter 16   Same-Sex Relationships 122

Chapter 17   Gender Roles and Expectations 128
             Transgender People 128
             Legal Inequality 129
             Property and Female Merchants 132
             Primogeniture and Valuing Boys 133
             Sex Ratios 134
             Valued Women 135

Abbreviations 137
Notes 139
Bibliography 160
Index 169

Kings of England in the Later Middle Ages

Henry III, reigned 1216 to 1272; son of King John and Isabelle of Angoulême; married Eleanor of Provence in 1236

Edward I, r. 1272 to 1307; son of Henry and Eleanor; married Leonor of Castile in 1254 and Marguerite of France in 1299

Edward II, r. 1307 to 1327; son of Edward and Leonor; married Isabella of France in 1308

Edward III, r. 1327 to 1377; son of Edward and Isabella; married Philippa of Hainault in 1328

Richard II, r. 1377 to 1399; son of Edward and Philippa's eldest son the Prince of Wales; married Anne of Bohemia in 1382 and Isabelle de Valois in 1396; childless

Henry IV, r. 1399 to 1413; son of Edward III and Philippa's son the Duke of Lancaster; married Mary de Bohun in 1394 and Juana of Navarre in 1403

Henry V, r. 1413 to 1422; son of Henry and Mary; married Katherine de Valois in 1420

Henry VI, r. 1422 to 1461 and 1470 to 1471; son of Henry and Katherine; married Marguerite of Anjou in 1445

Money

Twelve pennies (written d for *denarii*) made one shilling (s), and 20 shillings made one pound (£ or l for *librae*), i.e. 240d. Another unit of accounting was the mark, which was two-thirds of a pound and consisted of 160d or 13s and 4d. In the fourteenth century, a labourer typically earned 2d a day or £3 a year, and a master craftsman 6d a day.

Introduction

A few myths about medieval sexuality and sex lives are still current, or were until not too long ago: chastity belts, twelve-year-old girls routinely married off to men old enough to be their grandfathers, lords enjoying the *droit de seigneur* or the right to have sex with a bride on her wedding night, men penetrating their wives through a hole in a sheet for the purpose of procreation only, everyone being filthy and smelly with bad teeth, most weddings taking place in June because people had recently had their annual wash in May, and surely many more. It probably goes without saying that the reality is far more complex and interesting.

One major issue when writing about personal and intimate matters in medieval times is that diaries did not exist yet, and personal letters were few and far between, so it is extremely difficult to know for certain what people thought of their own sexuality, or how they experienced their love lives and sex lives. There were, of course, no newspapers or magazines until centuries later, and although many Middle English poems took courtly love and the yearning for an unattainable woman as a frequent theme, little literature on the matter of sex and intimacy exists from medieval England. There is vanishingly little evidence for masturbation or erotic fantasies, and although, of course, it is beyond all doubt that some medieval people were same-sex attracted, nobody yet identified themselves as gay, bi or straight. There were important cultural differences, e.g. men often shared their bed with another man. This was not necessarily sexual but was a way of honouring another person and showing that you trusted him not to murder you in your sleep.

Sex and Sexuality in Medieval England covers the later medieval period, from roughly 1250/70 to 1450/70, and aims to debunk a few myths about medieval sexuality and to educate and entertain!

Chapter 1

Appearance

Cleanliness

Before starting an account of the intimate lives of medieval people, can we determine what they might have looked like? For a start, and perhaps most importantly, it is extremely unlikely that they were anything like as dirty as the modern imagination might think. Certainly, the Middle Ages was an era long before the invention of power showers, and hot baths – which required the heating of large quantities of water on a fire, numerous containers to fill a bathtub large enough for a person to immerse themselves in, and much manpower to carry away and empty all the containers again – were far too labour-intensive for most people to bother with very often, if at all. This does not, however, mean that people did not wash and keep themselves clean. There was always a possibility to wash with water from a pitcher or basin, even if one could not immerse one's whole body in hot water. In his will of 1361, Humphrey de Bohun, Earl of Hereford, bequeathed a basin which he used for washing his head to his sister Margaret, Countess of Devon. Margaret herself left a 'pair of basins which were for washing the hands' of her late husband Hugh Courtenay to Exeter Cathedral in 1391.[1]

Alan Hacford of Norfolk, who worked as a chaplain in the 1320s, owned a 'brass dish for washing the head', worth 2d, and in the 1310s Katherine of Lincoln owned a 'basin with a washing-vessel' worth the large sum of 4s. An inventory of the goods belonging to the late London fishmonger Thomas Mockyng in 1373 included seven wash-bowls.[2] People also often washed in a stream or river, and sometimes took their lives into their hands while doing so; coroners' rolls reveal that a few people drowned while washing themselves. Robert Waddenho drowned while washing in the River Nene in 1301, Maud Reynald drowned while bathing in a marl pit in Naseby, Northamptonshire in 1309 or

1310, and sixteen-year-old John Redebourne drowned while bathing in the Houndsditch in London in 1337. A few unfortunate Londoners, including Henry Overestolte in 1340, drowned in the Thames while washing themselves.[3]

The three related texts about women's medicine known as the *Trotula* (meaning 'little Trota', a woman's name), written in Salerno in the twelfth century, were well-known in medieval England both in the original Latin and in Middle English translation.[4] The *Trotula* has a long section on how women should bathe and remove their body hair, and for washing one's hair, it recommends a shampoo of burnt vines, chaff of barley and liquorice wood. It includes tips on how a woman should wear cosmetics, which begins with an instruction that she should 'wash her face very well with French soap and warm water'.[5] The fifteenth-century *Boke of Nurture* includes instructions on how to prepare a bath for one's lord. A servant should hang 'sheets full of sweet herbs' from the roof, and ensure that five or six sponges to lean on were available, plus one large sponge to sit on and another under the feet. Using a basin containing hot water and fresh herbs, the lord's body was to be washed with a soft sponge and afterwards rinsed with warm rose water. The servant should dry him with a clean cloth as he stood on a foot-sheet, then fetch his socks and slippers and take him to bed. The *Boke* also contains instructions for medicinal baths. For 'ache', water as hot as the person could tolerate containing eighteen herbs including St John's wort, mallow, camomile and brown fennel, was recommended.[6]

Edward I's daughter Eleanor (1269–98), son Henry (1268–74) and nephew John of Brittany (1266–1334) were bathed regularly by their carers in childhood, and Spanish soap was purchased for the children. Medieval soap came in white, grey and black varieties and could be purchased by the loaf or cake. Eleanor and Henry's little brother Edward of Caernarfon, aged six, was bathed in 1290 while staying at Banstead in Surrey, and it cost 6d.[7] Edward I himself had running water in his tiled bathroom, controlled by gilt bronze taps, and his grandson Edward III had both hot and cold running water in several of his palaces.[8] Edward III's grandson and successor Richard II rebuilt the bathhouse at the royal residence of Langley in Hertfordshire, which had ten glazed windows, and built another luxurious bathhouse at his palace of Sheen with 2,000 painted tiles and large bronze taps for hot and cold water.[9] In his 1354 *Book of Holy Medicines*, Henry of

Appearance

Grosmont (*c.* 1310–61), first Duke of Lancaster, a cousin of Edward III and grandfather of Henry IV, described the benefits of a good bath which cleaned the body, and said that afterwards, he felt 'like a new man'. After the bath, Henry recommended that a person should 'sweat well' (*bien suer*). The *Trotula* also described a procedure that sounds exactly like a modern sauna.[10]

Clothes could also be washed in streams or rivers, and in London, there existed the *Lavenderebrigge*, located close to the modern Southwark Bridge. This word literally means 'Laundress's Bridge', though it was a wharf or jetty with steps down to the river where washerwomen worked. Washing clothes was usually a job done by women in late medieval England, though in the early 1300s John Tucke drowned in the village of Glinton (then in Northamptonshire, now in Cambridgeshire) while washing clothes in a stream. Although John's age is not given, it was possible that he was a child rather than a grown man.[11] The mayor and aldermen of London complained in 1417 that owners of 'certain wharves and stairs on the bank of the Thames' forced poor people who wished to wash and beat their clothes there to pay for the privilege and ordered them not to do so.[12] Noble households employed washerwomen, and in 1318, Amice Maure, Cristiane Scot, Annote Walisshe, 'dame Gonnore' and 'the wife of Simon Gawer' washed the clothes of the royal household. Edward IV's household ordinance of 1478 stated 'if ther be a quene in housholde, than there be women lauenders' (laundresses), and for the king himself, a servant was to purchase 'asmuch white sope [soap], gray and blak as can be thought reasonable'.[13]

Unpleasant smells, to the medieval mind, signified danger, corruption, spiritual uncleanliness, and death. Herbs and spices were, therefore, often used and scattered around to provide sweet smells.[14] Henry of Grosmont wrote in 1354 of his love of the aroma of expensive new cloth, flowers and rich food, and his shame at feeling involuntary revulsion for the stench of his comrades' wounds and the way poor, sick people smelled.[15] Even in an age long before modern dentistry, teeth might not always have been as decayed, rotten and smelly as we might think, given that few people had the chance to consume sugar regularly. When the remains of Bartholomew Burghersh, an English knight who died in 1369 in his late forties, were examined in 1961, he was found to have had a full set of teeth, albeit very worn.[16] For whitening teeth and for curing halitosis caused by rotted gums, the *Trotula* recommended a powder of cinnamon, clove, spikenard, mastic, frankincense, wormwood, crab foot, date pits and olives, to be rubbed onto the teeth and gums. The thirteenth-century physician Gilbertus Anglicus ('Gilbert the Englishman'), meanwhile, sensibly suggested drying one's teeth with a linen cloth after eating to ensure that no food stuck to them and rotted them.[17]

Clothing

Medieval manuscripts, such as the gorgeously illustrated Luttrell Psalter made in the first half of the fourteenth century, reveal how contemporaries dressed. Men in the early fourteenth century wore their hair to chin or shoulder level, parted in the middle and framing their face. A century later, the fashion had changed completely, and men wore their hair very short, cut up the back of the head. It is difficult to generalise about facial hair; some men had moustaches, others had bushy beards or goatee-style beards, while yet others preferred to be clean-shaven. Women wore their hair very long, and fourteenth-century noblewomen often wore their hair in plaits or braids twisted into coils and pinned at each side of their head, a style similar to that worn by Princess Leia. Blonde hair, pale skin and a certain plumpness or voluptuousness were considered desirable in women, as poet Geoffrey Chaucer's depiction of the great heiress Blanche of Lancaster in the 1360s makes apparent:

> She was bothe fair and bright...
> Right faire shuldres, and body long
> She hadde, and armes; every lith [limb]
> Fattish, flesshy, not greet therwith;
> Right whyte handes, and nayles rede [nails red],
> Rounde brestes; and of good brede [breadth]
> Hyr hippes were, a streight flat bake [back].[18]

Pale skin was prized as it signified wealth and privilege; most people worked outside all day, and only the wealthy were able to remain indoors and to have skin that was not tanned or damaged by the sun. To be 'fattish' and 'fleshy' in a world where few people had ample food also signified wealth. On the other hand, in his Miller's Tale, Chaucer describes the miller's beautiful and desirable young wife Alison thus: *As any wezele hir body gent and smal,* 'As any weasel, her body was

Appearance

graceful and slender'.[19] The meaning of this comparison to a weasel is much debated, but Chaucer surely meant to pay Alison a compliment and did not intend the 'slender' remark pejoratively.

Both women and men covered their heads, with hats, caps, hoods, coifs, or, in the case of women, headdresses or veils. The working men depicted in the Luttrell Psalter wear coifs or hoods pulled over their heads, and the long peak of the hood falls past their shoulders. Edward II in the 1320s owned a black hat lined with red velvet and decorated with butterflies made of pearls and a white hat lined with green velvet and decorated with gold trefoils.[20] When his wife Isabella of France moved to England in early 1308, her trousseau included two gold circlets and three hats or head-coverings adorned with rubies and emeralds, and Isabella's daughter-in-law Philippa of Hainault wore 'a hood made of brown scarlet studded with 154 stars of pearls and trimmed with gold'.[21] Two noblewomen depicted eating at a table in the Luttrell Psalter wear their hair pinned in coils at each side, with a narrow band of material around their head holding in place a diaphanous veil, which falls down their backs. The seal of Edward I's eldest granddaughter Eleanor, Lady Despenser (1292–1337), made in 1329, shows her wearing a floor-length gown and a simple veil, and the effigy of Eleanor's daughter-in-law Elizabeth, Lady Despenser, who died in 1359 and was buried in Tewkesbury Abbey in Gloucestershire, depicts her in a square headdress which must have been the height of contemporary fashion. Both the Luttrell Psalter and the effigy of Blanche, Lady Grandisson (d. 1347), in the church of St Bartholomew, Much Marcle, Herefordshire, show that fourteenth-century noblewomen often covered their neck, chin and the sides of their faces with a wimple.

When seventeen-year-old Constanza of Castile arrived in England in 1371, her new husband John of Gaunt, Duke of Lancaster, purchased almost 500 pearls to make a 'fret', i.e. a headdress of interlaced wire decorated with jewels, for her. Two years later, the duke bought two fillets, headbands also made of interlaced wire, for his daughters, thirteen-year-old Philippa and ten-year-old Elizabeth. Each had three balas rubies and twenty-eight pearls.[22] The effigy of John's mother Philippa of Hainault, Queen of England, in Westminster Abbey wears a reticulated headdress, where the hair was encased on either side of the head in bags made of gold or silver thread. Horned headdresses became fashionable in England in the early fifteenth century. Beatriz of

Portugal, Countess of Arundel, Surrey and Huntingdon, was buried with her first husband in 1439, and their extant effigies show the countess wearing a horned headdress of astonishing width and height, with material draped over the two points and her hair gathered in large coils at each side of her head and encased in jewelled hairnets. Headdresses called hennins, in the shape of a cone or steeple and often remarkably high, also became fashionable, while another popular horned style of the era was the bourrelet or escoffion, made from a thick padded roll of material. The *Trotula* recommended that noblewomen should wear musk, cloves, nutmeg or 'other sweet-smelling substances' in their hair, under their veil or head-covering, and also shared numerous recipes for colouring the hair blonde, black, or white. For whitening the hair, the authors recommended, not terribly helpfully, that women should 'catch as many bees as possible in a new pot and set it to burn'. The dead, burnt bees were to be mixed with oil and rubbed over the hair.[23]

Everyone, men and women of all ranks, wore hose, a kind of leggings, to cover their legs. During the blazingly hot, dry summer of 1326, Edward II bought linen cloth to make hose for the archers who formed his bodyguard, though in winter, hose would be made of wool or another thick material for warmth.[24] In the northern European climate, wearing thick clothes in winter assumed a great importance, and people often wore animal fur to keep warm. Miniver, very costly white or light grey fur made from the winter coat of the squirrel, was worn by wealthy noble or royal people. Other varieties of fur were 'budge' or lambskin, *scrimpyns* (cheap and poor quality furs), *roskyn* (fur of the squirrel in summer), *polan* (fur of the black squirrel), *stranglin* (fur of the squirrel around Michaelmas, 29 September) and *stradlynge* (fur of the squirrel between Michaelmas and winter). In 1324, a man's jerkin made of six pieces of otter skin cost 24d.[25]

Both men and women often wore *cotes* or tunics, *courtepies* or short jackets, *surcotes* or overtunics, *cotes hardies*, a long, fitted outer garment with long sleeves and sometimes hoods, which was buttoned or laced up the front, and, when the weather dictated, a *mantel* or cloak. Wills and other documents often used the phrase 'a robe of/with garments', which meant a complete set of clothes. One 'robe with three garments' consisted of a tunic, an overtunic and a cloak. Men wore shirts tied to their hose, and women wore floor-length gowns with long sleeves. 'Sideless surcoats' or over-gowns were very fashionable in the fourteenth century, with an undergown in a contrasting colour showcased by a large cut-out at each side. Medieval fashion could be as absurd and impractical as in later centuries; in the late 1300s, Richard II and his youthful male courtiers wore *cracowes*, soft shoes with toes so long that they had to be tied to the wearer's leg if he wished to be able to walk in them.

Medieval people were not free to dress however they wished to express themselves. In England, the first sumptuary laws, the official guidelines which dictated the clothes which different ranks of society were allowed to wear, date from Edward III's reign. Unofficially, however, they existed long before that, and it would always have been immediately obvious, from fabric, fur, embroidery, jewellery, and so on, where people stood in the strict social hierarchy of medieval England. In March 1322, when Edward II had his cousin Thomas, Earl of Lancaster beheaded outside Thomas's own castle at Pontefract in Yorkshire, he forced him to wear the striped cloth which the squires of Thomas's household wore. This was intended as a deliberate humiliation of a man of royal birth.

As an example of medieval sumptuary laws, knights with an annual income of under 200 marks and their families were not allowed to wear cloth worth more than six marks (960d), and women were not allowed to wear jewels except in their hair. Carters, cowherds and everyone else who worked on the land and did not have 40s of goods could wear nothing except russet or blanket cloth at 12d an ell (45 inches), and rope belts.[26] Russet cloth was coarse and either grey or black, and cost 12d or 12½d an ell in the 1320s. By way of contrast, the rich and colourful silken fabrics worn by those of much higher rank cost somewhere around 120d an ell.[27] As well as the sumptuary laws, in May 1327 Edward III ordained that 'no man or woman ... in England, Ireland or Wales, shall, after Christmas next, use cloth of his or her own buying which was not made in England, Ireland or Wales'.[28]

Geoffroi de Charny (c. 1300–56), a renowned French knight who spent time in England in the 1340s as a prisoner of war, composed three works on chivalry. He believed that women 'should pay more attention to their physical appearance and be more splendidly adorned' with jewels and ornaments than men. Charny warned, however, that excessive pride in one's dress could easily lead to a person forgetting God, and 'if you do not remember God, God will not remember you'.[29] Clothes were used to signal and to set apart women who were deemed 'disreputable' or 'of bad character'. A proclamation was made in London in 1281 that 'no woman of the town shall henceforth go to market nor into the highway out of her house with a hood furred with budge, whether it be of lamb or of conies [rabbit], upon pain of forfeiting her hood'. It went on to say that 'brewsters, nurses, other servants, and women of disreputable character' – why any of these groups of women were 'disreputable' was not explained – must not wear expensive miniver fur 'after the manner of reputable women'. In 1351, it was proclaimed in London that 'common lewd women' must not wear any garment lined with fur, sendal or samite cloth, 'or any other noble lining', either in winter or summer. The women were ordered to wear, both day and night, 'a hood of cloth of ray', i.e. striped cloth, so that everyone in the city, both residents and visitors, 'may have knowledge of what rank they are'. In 1381/82, it was once more 'ordained that common harlots and all women of bad character shall wear rayed [striped] hoods and use no manner of fur'.[30]

Chapter 2

Marriage (1)

Age at Marriage

One widespread modern misconception is that everyone in the Middle Ages married in childhood or early adolescence. This was indeed sometimes the case for those of royal and noble birth, boys as well as girls, such as Edward III's son Lionel of Antwerp, Duke of Clarence and Earl of Ulster. He was born on 29 November 1338, and married the heiress Elizabeth de Burgh, born 6 July 1332, on 15 August 1342 when he was only three years old and she was ten.[1] Edward III's brother-in-law David II of Scotland married Edward's sister Joan of the Tower on 17 July 1328 when Joan had just turned seven years old and David, born on 5 March 1324, was only four. Edmund Mortimer, born in February 1352 and heir to the earldom of March, married Philippa of Clarence, born in August 1355 as the only child of Lionel of Antwerp and Elizabeth de Burgh, in December 1358 when they were six and three respectively.[2]

Maud of Lancaster, one of the two co-heirs of her father the Earl of Derby and her grandfather the Earl of Lancaster and Leicester, was born on 4 April 1340 and married on 30 November 1344. Her husband was Ralph Stafford, heir to his grandfather the Earl of Gloucester and his father the future Earl of Stafford, and he was born not too long before 16 March 1339.[3] Ralph's younger brother Hugh Stafford was born sometime between 1342 and 1346 and married Philippa Beauchamp, daughter of the Earl of Warwick, in 1351.[4] Richard Neville, eldest son and heir of the Earl of Salisbury, married Anne Beauchamp, fourth daughter and ultimately the sole heir of the Earl of Warwick, in 1434 when he was six and she was eight; Anne's maternal grandparents Thomas Despenser and Constance of York had married in 1379 when Thomas was six and Constance about four or five. Edward I arranged the marriage of his youngest daughter Elizabeth of Rhuddlan in January 1285 when she was two and a half and her fiancé Jan, son and heir of the Count of Holland, was only a few months old. Nobles sometimes arranged betrothals for children who had not even been born, as Elizabeth Woodville, soon to become the queen of Edward IV, did in 1464 when she betrothed her son Thomas Grey to an as yet unborn daughter of William, Lord Hastings. Mere days after Robert Beyvill, heir to a landowning family in Huntingdonshire, was born in 1342, his parents' neighbour Walter Wastel stated 'half in jest' that Robert should one day marry Walter's daughter, born a few hours later. Walter was surprised when Robert's father Richard agreed that 'this should be done unless something better were found'.[5] Child-marriages almost always involved two children, and it was only very rarely the case that young girls were married off to much older men, another common modern misconception.

One notable exception, often cited, was the marriage of Margaret Beaufort and Edmund Tudor, Earl of Richmond, parents of Henry VII and grandparents of Henry VIII. Margaret was almost certainly born on 31 May 1443 and Edmund in c. 1430, and Margaret gave birth to Henry VII on 28 January 1457, which was only eight months after her thirteenth birthday and would mean that she conceived when she was still only twelve. Edmund was then in his mid-twenties. Margaret was the only legitimate child of John, Duke of Somerset and was also the heir of her wealthy great-uncle Henry, Cardinal Beaufort, and a custom known as the 'courtesy of England' gave a man who married an heiress an incentive to have a child with her as soon as possible. If the heiress died without any children by her husband, he had no claim to any part of her lands, which after her death would pass to her rightful heir by blood, usually an uncle or nephew or cousin. If, however, she gave birth to her husband's child and it lived long enough to take a breath – stillbirths did not count – the husband had the right to hold her entire estate for as long as he lived, even if his wife died many years before him.[6] There was little reason for men to marry and swiftly produce a child with women who were not heiresses, and the disturbingly early consummation of Margaret Beaufort and Edmund Tudor's marriage, while not unique (see Chapter 11 below), was an outlier.

Royal marriages of the Middle Ages can be seen as something akin to the merger of two mighty companies. They were usually arranged to end a war between two kingdoms, or to prevent a war occurring, or to cement an alliance against a third party. The marriage of fifteen-year-old

Marriage (1)

Lord Edward of England and twelve- or thirteen-year-old Doña Leonor of Castile was arranged in 1254 to prevent a war between Edward's father Henry III, who was Duke of Aquitaine in southern France as well as King of England, and Leonor's brother Alfonso X of Castile, who wished to invade and annex Aquitaine, his neighbour to the north. Edward and Leonor's son Edward of Caernarfon, later Edward II, was betrothed to Isabella of France in 1299 to finalise a peace settlement between Edward I and Isabella's father Philip IV, who had gone to war in 1294. Isabella was about four years old; Edward was fifteen and it was his fourth betrothal; the first had taken place in 1289 when he was five.

Marriages among the nobility almost always had far more to do with acquiring land, making alliances and gaining powerful in-laws than with love. Sir John Neville, brother of the Earl of Westmorland, openly admitted in 1446 that he wished to marry Margaret, dowager Duchess of Somerset, because of the rich dower lands she held, though he did also state that he was 'induced by the ardour of a singular affection'. Duchess Margaret was apparently less enamoured of Neville, and married Lionel, Baron Welles instead. Undeterred, Neville married Anne Holland, daughter of the Duke of Exeter and widow of his own nephew, though he claimed that Anne's first marriage had never been consummated. In 1452, Neville talked of his and his wife's 'ardour of mutual affection', but admitted that he had really married her 'in order that [he] might acquire certain manors belonging to the said Anne' from her marriage to his nephew.[7] John Neville was unusual only in being so open about his desire for lands, though the desire was almost universal. In 1292, Edward I negotiated an extraordinarily favourable marriage for his nephew Thomas of Lancaster (b. c. 1277/78) with Alice de Lacy (b. 1281), sole heir of the wealthy Lacy and Longespee families. Thomas and his Lancaster heirs would keep all of Alice's lands even if the couple had no surviving children, as indeed happened.[8]

Another reason for noble marriages was to 'end enmity' between two families. Henry III's half-brother William de Valence, Earl of Pembroke, and Sir Henry Hastings stood on opposite sides of the baronial wars of the 1260s. To 'settle their enmity', the families arranged the marriage of Valence's daughter Isabel and Hastings' son John sometime before March 1269. John Hastings was six at the time, Isabel probably younger, and they married sometime after July 1275 and had at least five children together.[9] In 1330, William de Bohun, later Earl of Northampton, was one of the men who helped his cousin Edward III arrest Roger Mortimer, Earl of March, co-ruler of the king's mother Isabella during the young king's minority. Roger was subsequently hanged. Five years later, William married Elizabeth Badlesmere, widow of Roger's son Edmund, 'to put an end to enmities between the two families'.[10]

Further down the social scale, there was little incentive for child-marriages, and most of the common people of England, with a few exceptions, married in their late teens or twenties, sometimes in their thirties. It seems from the evidence we have that women usually married husbands who were a few years their senior, and that it was common for women to marry in their late teens or at the start of their twenties. Agnes Twomer was born c. 1331/32 as the daughter of a tanner in London and married the saddler Henry Myre in 1349 when she was seventeen or eighteen, and Isabel Hakeneye, youngest child of the London woolmonger Richard Hakeneye, married the fishmonger William Olneye in 1362 when she was twenty. Alice Helpestone of London married Thomas Wythe in 1356 when she was nineteen, and her sister Joan married Henry Piryman in 1364 when she was eighteen; Margery Neketon married Alexander Bedyk in late 1377 or early 1378 when she was eighteen; Alice atte Berne was born in or before June 1347 and married William West in October 1366; and Joan Ussher was born c. November 1375 and married Walter Kyng in May 1393.[11] Rohese, eldest daughter of Thomas Romeyn, Mayor of London in 1309/10, was born c. 1286, married John Burford before December 1312, and gave birth to their son James, one of their three children, in c. 1320 when she was about thirty-four.[12] Alice, one of the three daughters of Robert Ram, was born in Kent on 28 October 1349, married Robert Freman when she was eighteen, and gave birth to her eldest son (not necessarily her first child) around Christmas 1370 at age twenty-one.[13] Men tended to be a few years older when they wed. To give just a handful of examples of many, John atte Well was thirty-seven when he married Agnes atte Lynde in Ifield, Sussex on 18 September 1358, John Brampton was twenty-seven when he married his wife Isabel in Morpeth, Northumberland on 2 February 1372, Richard Crawecestre was twenty-nine when he married 'the daughter of William Urde' in Newcastle-upon-Tyne on 23 April 1389, and Thomas Yardley was thirty-six when he married Joan in Coventry on 1 June 1409. Richard Casewell, an unusually young bridegroom, was sixteen when he married Joan Beaumeys in Tarrington, Herefordshire on 8 September 1345.[14]

Marriage (1)

The two daughters of Robert Lambrouk of South Petherton, Somerset, both married in June 1380, and their husbands were John Peny, aged twenty-seven, and John Warmwell, aged twenty-three; the women's ages, and indeed their names, are not known.[15]

There were, however, some exceptions, usually where property or valuable goods were involved, when people of common birth married as children or in their early teens. In 1315, London resident Simon Burgh and his wife Maud arranged the marriage of Maud's daughter Agnes, whose father was Maud's first husband John Laurence, to Simon's son Thomas from his first marriage. Thomas Burgh was ten at the time and Agnes Laurence was eight, and would inherit property worth forty marks (6,400d) annually from her late father when she came of age. Simon wished his son to benefit financially from marrying his stepsister, and Maud enthusiastically went along with the idea. Simon and Maud had already had the banns of marriage published and purchased wedding clothes and food for the feast, but concerned adults brought the matter to the attention of the mayor and aldermen of London, who removed Agnes Laurence from her mother's and stepfather's custody.[16] Another example is John Garton, an orphan, who was already married to the unnamed daughter of John Bas in November 1376, although he was only nine years old. John Hatfeld, a well-off chandler of London, died in c. September/October 1363, and left lands, tenements and numerous household goods to his daughter Dionise. He also specified that his fellow chandler Robert Kyng should have custody of Dionise until she turned sixteen. By November 1364, however, though she was only fourteen and a half, Dionise had already married Richard Claverynge, a draper of London. Margaret Godyn was born in 1388 and married Roger Lughtburghe in or shortly before December 1402, when she was fourteen; her inheritance from her father Henry was a substantial £120. In 1250, fifteen-year-old Isabel Ford, granddaughter and heir of Robert Muschaump, was 'married to a boy named Adam Wyginton, aged thirteen or fourteen'.[17]

It was usually the case that the medieval bridegroom was older than the bride, though there were exceptions, such as Lionel of Antwerp and Elizabeth de Burgh in 1342. Lionel's niece Elizabeth of Lancaster married John Hastings, heir to the earldom of Pembroke, in June 1380 when she was sixteen or seventeen and he, born in November 1372, was just seven.[18] Elizabeth's half-sister Catalina of Lancaster was born sometime between early June 1372 and late March 1373, and in September 1388 married Enrique III, King of Castile, born in October 1379. John Arundel was the fourth child of the Earl of Arundel (d. 1376) and his second wife Eleanor of Lancaster (d. 1372), who married in February 1345. John was married as a child in c. 1357/59 to the heiress Eleanor Maltravers, who was some years his senior and born c. 1344, and the eldest of their seven children was born in late 1364 when John is unlikely to have been older than about fourteen.[19] Philippa Arundel (d. 1399), a granddaughter of the earls of Arundel (d. 1376) and Salisbury (d. 1344), gave birth to her eldest child around 1367/70, became a grandmother in 1393, and cannot have been born later than the early or mid-1350s. In 1398 she married her second husband Sir John Cornwall, who was much her junior, perhaps twenty years younger; he did not die until 1443.[20]

In noble marriages where the wife was a few years older than her husband, she had to wait until he grew up in order to enjoy intimacy; an unwritten rule dictated that men who married a much younger wife had the freedom to have outside interests while they waited for their wives to reach maturity, but noble and royal women were strictly enjoined to remain virgins. Elizabeth of Lancaster, married to a boy almost a decade her junior, was unable to wait. In June 1386, six years after her wedding, when she was twenty-two or twenty-three and her husband was still only thirteen, her marriage was hastily annulled so that she could marry Sir John Holland instead, almost certainly because she was already pregnant by him. Some couples who wed in childhood rejected their marriages when they were older; see 'Disputed and Unhappy Marriages' in Chapter 5. An inquisition was held in Yorkshire in January 1430 to determine whether John Salveyn, who inherited several manors in the county from his parents George and Elizabeth and had married Joan Gray twelve years earlier when he was only ten, had consented to marrying her and had done so while of sound mind. The finding was that he had indeed wed Joan of his own free will, and that the couple were still married and had a daughter, Joan the younger.[21]

In 1476, in London, Margaret Pounde was allowed to enter into her inheritance from her late father when she either turned sixteen or married. In the same era, Joan Swift was allowed to inherit her late father's property either when she turned fifteen or when she married.[22] In London in the second half of the fifteenth century, fifteen or sixteen was considered a reasonable and mature age for a girl to marry and to engage in regular sexual relations with her husband; twelve was not.

Weddings

Weddings were not always celebrated in a church or a chapel, and when they were, they took place at the door rather than inside. The Prologue narrated by Geoffrey Chaucer's famous Wife of Bath in his *Canterbury Tales*, written in the late fourteenth century, makes this clear: 'Housbondes at chirche dore I have had fyve'.[23] Isabella Pledour of London stated in the late 1380s, when trying to annul her marriage, that she had married Richard Lyons 'at the door of St Mary de Stanynge Church in Aldrichesgate' (St Mary Staining, Aldersgate) in 1363. Simon Clathorpe and Alice Norman married at the door of the church in Bilsby, Lincolnshire, on 20 July 1315. Ralph Adrien, an Italian who lived in England and died in early 1286, stated in his will that he had endowed his wife Jacobina with his London house at the church door when he married her. John Flete, a cap-maker of Ludgate in London, said in early 1280 that he had endowed his wife Cassandra with two houses in the parish of St Martin at the church door when they wed. The Latin expression *ad ostium ecclesie* is also sometimes translated as 'in the porch of the church'.[24] After the ceremony, the newlyweds and their guests went inside the church to hear Mass.

Weddings sometimes took place at the same time and in the same church as baptisms. On 10 August 1339, Robert and Emma Whit married in a church in Laxton, Nottinghamshire at the same time that John Bekeryng was baptised there, and the wedding of Walter More and Margaret Keynes was conducted in the church of Glanvilles Wootton in Dorset on 2 May 1362, while the baptism of Nicholas Toner was taking place nearby.[25] The reading of marriage banns on three occasions prior to a wedding was essential, as otherwise, any children of the marriage would be deemed illegitimate. In 1432 in Norfolk, William Leche and Agnes Childe's children John and Alice were determined to be illegitimate because 'marriage banns were never read for William and Agnes', and thus they had no right to the property of their older half-sister Sybil. Pope Clement VI issued a dispensation for Simon Leyk and Margaret Vaux in 1351 'to remain in the marriage which they contracted without banns', and declared their children legitimate.[26] Banns of marriage between Madoc ap Madoc and his wife Sybil were published in their parish church in Welshpool on Sunday, 25 April 1361, and they married on Thursday 6 May following. On 7 January 1395, George Percy and Alice Whetely of Applegarth in Yorkshire 'contracted matrimony' and subsequently married after the banns had been read, and on 23 April 1388, twenty-seven-year-old William Hommedenys of Wiltshire 'contracted to marry a woman of Ramsbury called Alice Westende', went to his local parish church, and asked the chaplain to publish the banns. John Smolt of Little Wakering, Essex 'affianced himself to' Margaret Parker on 1 January 1313, and married her around 2 February that year.[27]

The medieval wedding ceremony itself was remarkably similar to the modern ceremony. Rings were exchanged; Edward I's fourteen-year-old daughter Elizabeth of Rhuddlan was given a gold ring by her twelve-year-old bridegroom, Jan, Count of Holland, in early 1297.[28] The wedding of John Giffard and Aubrey Camville took place in the church of Cookhill Priory in Worcestershire, on c. Wednesday, 21 August 1241, sometime between 'the third and ninth hour of the day', i.e. nine a.m. to mid-afternoon. Brother Richard, a canon of Studley, officiated at this wedding of two children: they were both about eight years old and had been betrothed since they were about four, and Aubrey 'was taller than the husband'. John said 'I take thee, Aubrey, to my lawful wife, to have and to hold all the days of my life', and she answered with the same words. John took a ring from Brother Richard's hand and said 'With this ring I thee wed, and with my body and goods I thee honour'. Brother Richard then celebrated Mass, and the newly-married child-couple walked or rode at the head of a procession and enjoyed a feast.[29] After their wedding in July 1291, John and Emma Frie of Pitton in Wiltshire walked at the head of a 'great company' of wedding guests, though sadly one local resident, William Champeneys, was 'very abusive' to them and John hit him over the head with a stick, somewhat marring the happy occasion.[30]

In the liturgy of the medieval Church, recorded in Middle English, the bridegroom said:

> I, N., take the, N., to my wedded wyf, to haue and to holde fro this day forwarde, for better for wors, for richer for pouerer, in sykenesse and in hele, tyll dethe vs departe, if holy churche it woll ordeyne, and thereto y plight the my trouthe.

The bride said the same, substituting *housbonde* for *wyf*, with the addition of the following words before *tyll dethe vs departe*: *to be bonere and buxum in bedde and atte borde*.[31] *Bonere* and *buxum* both meant obedient or meek.

Wedding Customs

In the early fourteenth century, there was a popular custom to throw pennies over a bridal couple, or least over wealthier bridal couples, to bring them luck. The money was gathered up and distributed to the poor as alms, or picked up from the ground by poor people themselves. Edward II donated over £7 in coins at the wedding of his niece Margaret de Clare and the Earl of Cornwall in November 1307, and in February 1321 gave out £2 at the wedding of his great-niece Isabella Despenser and the Earl of Arundel's son Richard, a child-couple of eight and seven years old respectively. By the early fifteenth century, weddings were often celebrated by playing *foteball(e)*, i.e. football, and, less happily for modern sensibilities, by *cokthresshyng* or 'cock-thrashing', throwing sticks or lashing at tethered birds while wearing a blindfold. In 1409, Henry IV forbade 'the levying of money for the games called *foteball* and *cokthresshyng* on occasion of marriages'. Eight men in London entered into a bond on 4 March 1409 that 'none of them would in future collect money for a football or money called *cok sylver* for a cock, hen, capon, pullet or other bird' to *thresshe* in the streets and lanes of London. To celebrate a wedding held in Romney, Kent in 1257, a crowd gathered to watch a group of men tilting at the quintain, and at an unspecified 'game' held to celebrate the wedding of Nicholas Hastings and his unnamed wife in Westmorland in 1286, Robert Appelleby killed Nicholas with an arrow because he 'much loved' Nicholas's wife. Playing football or another type of ball-game to mark a wedding might have been a long-standing tradition: during a wedding procession in Yorkshire in 1268, a local resident asked one of the wedding guests for a ball (*pelota* in the Latin original), 'which it is the custom to give'.[32]

In 1241, John Giffard and Aubrey Camville both wore green robes when they married, and in September 1410, twenty-five-year-old Matthew Honorre of Odell in Bedfordshire had himself a silver belt 'studded with bells' made for his wedding.[33] Edward I's eighteen-year-old daughter Joan of Acre bought a headdress made partly of gold with rubies and emeralds and a matching belt in Paris for her wedding to the Earl of Gloucester on 30 April 1290.[34] Maurice, Lord Berkeley, badly wounded during the battle of Poitiers in 1356 and an invalid for the remaining twelve years of his life, was unable to travel from Gloucestershire to Buckinghamshire to attend his fourteen-year-old son Thomas's wedding to Margaret Lisle in 1367, but had himself a robe of cloth-of-gold made for the occasion. The bridegroom himself wore satin and scarlet cloth with a silver belt, while the three knights and twenty-three squires who accompanied him wore striped cloth furred with miniver.[35]

The *droit de seigneur* or 'lord's right', sometimes rendered in Latin as *ius primae noctis* or 'right of the first night', is the supposed entitlement of a medieval lord to have sex with, or rape, rather, the bride of one of his vassals on her wedding night. It is now universally assumed to be a myth, its appearance in the film *Braveheart* notwithstanding, and was something discussed over the centuries by several European writers who talked about it as a custom that had supposedly happened in earlier, less enlightened eras, but now did not. Another ridiculous and inaccurate alleged 'fact' often shared online states that medieval people married in June because May was the only time of year they washed, and therefore they still smelt relatively fresh. In addition, we are told, brides carried a bouquet of flowers to conceal their body odour. This is absolute nonsense. Weddings have indeed always been common in England in June because of the improving weather, but people in the Middle Ages married all year round, and sometimes in the depths of winter. Geoffrey and Lecia Catteworth married near Mears Ashby, Northamptonshire on Tuesday, 7 January 1276; Christine Ewfowle and Thomas Oketon married in Hawkedon, Suffolk on Tuesday, 25 November 1382; John and Margery Woghere married in East Grinstead, Sussex on Friday, 13 January 1402; and John Scolmayster, aged twenty-seven, married his wife Christine in Devon in the morning of Thursday, 18 January 1403.[36] As Melissa Snell points out, popular months for weddings in medieval England were January, October and November, 'when the harvest was past and the time for planting had not yet arrived'. Furthermore, late autumn and winter was the time of year when animals were slaughtered, so meat was available for wedding feasts.[37] Royal weddings also often took place in winter. Henry III and Eleanor of Provence married on 14 January 1236; their grandson Edward II married Isabella of France on 25 January 1308; Edward and Isabella's son Edward III married

Marriage (1)

Philippa of Hainault on c. 24/25 January 1328; Edward and Philippa's grandson Richard II married Anne of Bohemia on 20 January 1382; and another of their grandsons, Henry IV, married his second wife Juana of Navarre on 7 February 1403.

After a wedding, the guests would enjoy a feast with wine. The types of wine usually drunk in late medieval England were Gascon, i.e. red; Rhenish, i.e. white; or sweet, dessert wines called osey, tyre, bastard, romeney, clarrey or clary, malvesy or malmsey, or hippocras.[38] The banquet held in Winchester in February 1403 to celebrate Henry IV's wedding to Juana of Navarre, dowager Duchess of Brittany, represents the ultimate in medieval wedding feasts, and cost over £522. Guests dined on cygnets, venison, pullets, partridges, woodcock, quails, pears in syrup, custards, fritters, subtleties decorated with crowns and eagles, a cake in the shape of panthers, and much more.[39]

Present and Future Vows

Sponsalia per verba de presenti, 'betrothal by present vows', meant an exchange of promises made in the present, e.g. 'I, John, take thee, Joan, to be my lawful wedded wife'. Exchanging such vows made a marriage legal, even if they were taken in secret, without witnesses, and without any permission that might be required. Consummation made the marriage binding, though if it remained unconsummated, the marriage was still legal and could not be dissolved unless one spouse entered a monastery or if the pope granted a dispensation to dissolve it.[40] In 1319, Don Jaume, eldest son and heir of Jaume II of Aragon in Spain (r. 1291–1327), married Doña Leonor, daughter of the late Fernando IV of Castile (r. 1295–1312). Jaume refused to take a full part in the wedding ceremony or to consummate the marriage afterwards, and, renouncing his claim to his father's throne, announced his intention to become a monk. The marriage was soon annulled, aided by the fact that Leonor was only twelve, and a few years later she married Jaume's younger brother Alfonso and became queen-consort of Aragon.[41]

Sponsalia per verba de futuro meant when a couple promised to marry each other in the future. These vows did constitute an obligation to wed but not an indissoluble marriage as present vows did, and the promise could be dissolved under various conditions, including if one party took present vows with somebody else, or became a heretic, an apostate or a leper. A promise to wed in the future could also simply be dissolved if both parties consented.[42] One fourteenth-century case of *sponsalia per verba di futuro* was that of Joan Brereley and Thomas Bakester of York. Thomas told Joan, according to two witnesses, 'Joan, if you wish to wait until the end of my apprenticeship, I wish to take you as my wife'. Thomas, however, married another woman, Margaret Sandeshend, who six years later sued Thomas and Joan in a divorce action on the grounds of their pre-contract. After William Cardunvill of Hampshire died in 1254, an inquisition found that he had 'solemnly espoused at the church door one Alice' sixteen years earlier, and that the couple had several children together, of whom only four-year-old Richard still lived. Another woman named Joan, however, had a twenty-four-year-old son, also Richard, with William Cardunvill, and 'claimed the said William as her husband in Court Christian by a promise given to her', i.e. that he had sworn to wed her before he wed Alice. The jury found that, although William and Alice's marriage was therefore probably invalid, Joan was never rightfully 'espoused at the church door', and they were uncertain as to which of William's two sons named Richard should be his heir.[43]

It was possible to wed by proxy, i.e. two people in different locations nominated representatives to go through the wedding ceremony for them until they could marry in person. On the feast day of St Valentine, 14 February 1387, Edward III's granddaughter Philippa of Lancaster married King João of Portugal in the Portuguese cathedral of Porto, and they had first been married by proxy twelve days earlier, before the necessary papal dispensation for the marriage arrived. João Rodrigues de Sá stood in for King João.[44]

Chapter 3

Marriage (2)

Clandestine Marriages and Bigamy

The long-lived Margery Despenser (c. 1398–1478) was the daughter and heir of Philip Despenser and Elizabeth Tibetot, and inherited lands in five counties from her parents. Her marriage to John, Lord Ros (b. 1396) of Helmsley in Yorkshire was arranged in 1404 when they were both children. John was killed fighting in France in March 1421, leaving no children, and before 2 April 1423, Margery married her second husband without the necessary royal permission. He was Roger Wentworth of Yorkshire, and he was a mere squire and not even his father's eldest son, whereas Margery was of noble birth and an heiress. Pope Eugene IV declared in 1436 that Margery and Roger had contracted marriage lawfully, 'consummated it and had offspring, but could not have the marriage solemnised before the church after the custom of the country because, being unequal in nobility, they feared that scandals might arise among their kinsmen and friends'. Eugene declared that Margery and Roger's marriage was valid and their children legitimate. The government of the underage Henry VI pardoned the couple on 25 June 1423 for marrying without a royal licence, and fined them £1,000.[1] In 1469, Margery Paston, from a landowning family of some distinction, wed Richard Calle, her parents' bailiff. Her disgruntled family subsequently kept the couple apart until it became clear and undeniable that they had married clandestinely and were indeed husband and wife. During the period of forced separation, Richard wrote to Margery about 'the gret bonde of matrymonye that is made betwix vs, and also the greete loue that hath be, and I trust yet is, betwix vs, and as on my parte neuer gretter'.[2]

Clandestine marriages could cause problems for any children of the marriage: Pope John XXII had to issue a dispensation for John Hale in 1328, because Hale, born out of wedlock, had wrongly 'believ[ed] that by the subsequent clandestine marriage of his father and mother he was legitimated'. Eugene IV dealt with the case of Elizabeth Herderston of Norfolk in 1434. She admitted that she 'contracted espousals' with an unnamed man but 'without copulation', and at the urging of her family and friends, subsequently contracted marriage with another man *per verba di presenti* and did consummate this one, and had several children with him. Eugene absolved her from excommunication. In the early 1400s, Thomas Motte of the diocese of Norwich married a woman by *verba de presenti* 'clandestinely and without subsequent cohabitation', but afterwards contracted marriage with another woman also by *verba de presenti* 'publicly before the church' and had children with her. His first wife also married again, and by 1438 had lived with her second husband for more than thirty years. Eugene IV absolved both Thomas and his unnamed first wife from the sentence of excommunication, and ordered them to give generous alms to the poor as penance and to remarry their current spouses.[3]

Edward III issued a statute in 1344 declaring that cases of bigamy would be sent to the 'spiritual court', and in the Middle Ages, it was an offence dealt with by ecclesiastical rather than secular courts.[4] In 1443, Geoffrey Taillour of Devizes in Wiltshire was found to have committed bigamy by being married to Agnes White and Agnes Guphey at the same time. Geoffrey protested that his first wife died before he married his second. In August 1363, William Gernoun of Lindsey in Lincolnshire was imprisoned while the Bishop of Lincoln's court tried to determine whether his marriage to Katherine Alford was bigamous or not.[5] In or before 1469, Margery Chawei of London contracted marriage *per verba de presenti* with Thomas Mone, and while he was still alive contracted another marriage with *per verba de presenti* with William Thwaytys of Sussex, and cohabited with him. The case was referred to the pope.[6] Determining true cases of bigamy in the Middle Ages, i.e. simultaneous marriage to two or more spouses, is not aided by the contemporary habit of describing a person's second marriage after the death of his/her first spouse as 'bigamy' as well; in short, the concept of bigamy had a wider application in the Middle Ages than to us.[7] Confusingly, the word 'bigamy' was also used when a man was a clerk, i.e. had taken minor orders in the Church, but also married a woman. In 1414, the pope dealt with John Boghe, a 'married clerk of the diocese of Exeter', who had committed 'bigamy by marrying a widow, now dead'. Roger Aspeden, a married man, was imprisoned in Lancashire in 1378 'because of bigamy alleged against him after he claimed ... to be a clerk'.[8]

Marriage Rights

Under the feudal system of medieval England, those who held land directly from the king were called tenants in chief. Special rules applied to such people, including a provision that when they died, the king automatically became the guardian of their heir and owned the rights to the heir's marriage. Widows of tenants in chief took an oath not to marry again without the king's permission, and numerous entries in the chancery rolls along the lines of 'Licence for Eleanor, late the wife of Edmund Gascelyn, tenant in chief, to marry whomever she will of the king's allegiance' can be seen. The licence almost always had to be paid for, and the amount depended on the widow's income: Alice, whose late husband William Torel owned a few houses and meadows in Essex, only had to pay £2 in 1289, while Eleanor Berkeley, whose son John Arundel (b. 1408) was heir to the earldom of Arundel, paid £100 in 1423.[9] In 1357, Edward III ordered an official in Hampshire to investigate 'as to what widows have married without the king's licence after the death of their husbands, his tenants, whom, at what time and how much the marriage of each was worth, because the king is informed that some widows of tenants in chief have married without licence'. Edward's grandfather Edward I told officials in November 1298 to investigate Margaret, widow of Robert Valle, who 'refused to take an oath that she would not marry without the king's licence'. Her dower lands were confiscated.[10]

If the widow of a tenant in chief did not pay for a licence to remarry, the king often sold the rights to her second marriage. Margaret Basset lost her husband Sir Edmund Stafford in or soon before July 1308, and her brother Sir Ralph Basset of Drayton bought her marriage rights for 100 marks (£66.66). Margaret, however, married her second husband Thomas Pype before 26 August 1308 without the consent of the king or her brother, and Edward II confiscated her lands as punishment.[11] Joan Oreby (b. c. 1351), heir of the Oreby family, married Henry, Lord Percy (b. c. 1321) in 1365, and was widowed on c. 19 May 1368 a few weeks after she gave birth to their daughter Mary Percy. Edward III granted

Joan's marriage rights to Richard Stury on 29 July 1368, just ten weeks after she lost her husband.[12] Women often, however, had more choice regarding their second husband than this system may indicate. Edward II granted permission in 1326 for William Braose's widow Isabel to marry Simon Montbreton if she wished, 'but if she will not, she shall remain the king's widow, in the same condition that she is now, and may not marry any other without his licence'. Isabel did not marry Montbreton. Ten years later, Edward III gave the Earl of Warwick's brother John Beauchamp permission to marry the Earl of Hereford's widow Margaret, 'if she will marry him'. Margaret did not wish to; Beauchamp died unmarried, and Margaret preferred to live a religious life in widowhood. She went on a long journey to Santiago de Compostela and 'other holy places of pilgrimage in foreign parts' in 1344.[13] Many women took vows of chastity to avoid a second (or third) marriage; see Chapter 6 below.

Although men usually owned the rights to their own marriage when they came of age at twenty-one, they did not always have a great deal more choice than women regarding their spouse, and when they did, sometimes had to pay for the privilege. In July 1403, Henry IV granted the Earl of Arundel, Thomas Fitzalan, permission to 'marry whom he please' in exchange for a payment of 2,000 marks (£1,333.33). In 1405, however, Arundel agreed to the king's request, or demand, that he marry Beatriz, illegitimate daughter of Henry's brother-in-law King João of Portugal, to strengthen the bond between the two kingdoms. João begged Henry not to force his 'son' Arundel to pay the huge sum he owed.[14] Edward II offered the marriage of the late Earl of Cornwall's four-year-old daughter and heir Joan Gaveston, his own great-niece, to his eighteen-year-old ward Thomas Wake in 1316, but Wake wed the Earl of Lancaster's niece Blanche of Lancaster, who was much closer to his own age, instead. He had to pay a huge fine, probably £1,000, to the king. The government of the child-king Henry VI imposed a fine of £2,000 on John de Vere, Earl of Oxford (1408-62), for marrying Elizabeth Howard in 1425 without a royal licence and for refusing a suitable marriage offered to him. During Lent in 1352, Thomas Staple of Southwark offered his twenty-year-old ward John Amory of Leicestershire (b. November 1331) a choice between two brides: Alice Cleet of Berkshire or Isabel St Albans of Surrey. John 'utterly refused both, and of his own accord' married Eleanor Baryngton instead. An inquiry ordered by Edward III found that Thomas Staple had lost £200 from John's marriage, and

Marriage (2)

John acknowledged that he owed Thomas this amount. After he came of age in 1301, John Pavely of Somerset had to acknowledge a fine to his former guardian William Welles for refusing a marriage which Welles offered to him during his minority, and the lands he had inherited were withheld from him until he paid it in 1303. In 1350, Richard Pyjon of Pulborough in Sussex, aged thirty-nine, was forced by an ecclesiastical court to marry Joan atte Melle, who had a twenty-two-year-old son from her first marriage. An annoyed Richard stated that it was 'adjudged by law that he should have her to wife against his will'.[15]

Tenants in chief often broke the rule and married without the king's permission, which usually resulted in a fine and temporary seizure of lands and goods. Sir Hugh Despenser and the widowed Isabella Chaworth, née Beauchamp, married in or soon before December 1285, and had to admit liability to pay a fine of 2,000 marks to Edward I. The king confiscated their lands and goods and had made a profit of £400 from them by the time he returned them in January 1287, and let the couple off the rest of the fine.[16] Hugh and Isabella's daughter Isabella, Lady Hastings, married her third husband Ralph Monthermer in 1318 without a licence and was fined 1,000 marks, though never paid it.[17] Edmund Beaufort, the future Duke of Somerset, and Eleanor Beauchamp, widowed Lady Ros, married without permission sometime before 21 October 1434. They were finally pardoned on 7 March 1438 'for intermarrying without the king's licence' and excused from having to pay the due fine.[18]

The king often sold the marriage rights of a tenant in chief's heir or heiress, and the purchaser almost inevitably arranged the heir's marriage to a member of his or her family. Occasionally, however, the purchaser himself wed the heiress: in 1409, Henry IV sold the marriage of Agnes Battyng of Rye in Sussex, heir of her late father John, to Thomas Knyght, 'to the end that he may marry her himself'.[19] The sale of a marriage often included the provision that 'if the said heir dies during his minority unmarried, [the purchaser] shall have the marriage of the next heir if a minor, and so from heir to heir'. Juliana Leybourne (1303/4–67), was the heir of her father Sir Thomas (d. 1307) and of her grandfather William, Lord Leybourne, who became Juliana's guardian after his son's death. When Lord Leybourne died in 1310, Edward II sold Juliana's marriage to Aymer de Valence, Earl of Pembroke, who had no children of his own and arranged her marriage to his nephew and co-heir John,

Lord Hastings. Joan Verdon was born in August 1303, and lost her mother Maud Mortimer in 1312 and her father Sir Theobald Verdon in 1316. Joan and her sisters Elizabeth (b. c. 1306/07) and Margery (b. 1310), and their half-sister Isabella (b. 1317), were the Verdon heirs. Sir William Montacute (d. 1319) acquired Joan's marriage rights shortly after her father died, and she wed his eldest son John Montacute, born c. 1299, on 28 April 1317. John died mere months later, before 14 August 1317, and in February 1318 Joan married her second husband, Thomas Furnival. She was still only fourteen and a half years old when she married for the second time, though her first son was not born until June 1322, when she was almost nineteen.[20]

Gilbert de Clare, Earl of Gloucester, paid 1,000 marks (£666.66) in 1311 for the rights to the marriage of fourteen-year-old Robert, son and heir of the recently deceased Adam Welle. The earl, however, was killed at the Battle of Bannockburn in 1314 before he arranged a marriage for Robert, and the young man died still unmarried in August 1320.[21] In 1379, Henry Asty paid twenty marks to Richard II for the marriage of William, son and heir of the late Joan Bulneys, and in 1391, Sir Ralph Neville paid £100 for the marriage of Walter Heron's heir and £50 for the marriage of Robert Horsle's heir. Twenty years later, the wealthy Neville (now Earl of Westmorland) paid the massive sum of £2,000 to Henry IV for the marriage of John Mowbray, Earl of Nottingham and future Duke of Norfolk, one of the most important noblemen in the country. He married John to his daughter Katherine.[22] Edward II sold the marriages of the sisters Margery and Margaret Foliot, aged about twelve and eleven and heirs of their late brother Richard, to Isabella, Lady Hastings and Sir Ralph Camoys for £200 each in 1325. Margery Foliot married Isabella's son Hugh Hastings and Margaret married Ralph's son John Camoys.[23] In 1273, the marriage of Robert Exemue's widow Iseult was worth £14, in 1388 the marriage of Elizabeth, seven-year-old daughter and heir of Thomas Playce of Yorkshire, was worth £300, and in 1415 the marriage of twenty-year-old William Yonge, heir to his father's manor of Throckley in Northumberland, was worth £5. The marriage of Alice, underage daughter of the late London fishmonger Robert Fourneux, was worth £44 in 1363, and the marriage of Margaret, daughter of Henry Godyn, was worth £120 in 1402. In 1258, the marriage of Beatrice, widow of William Coroner, was 'worth 100*s* [£5] only, because she is much burdened with debts and the costs of her sons, and is beyond the age of childbearing'.[24]

Marriage (2)

An inquisition was held in Newcastle-upon-Tyne in 1426 to determine whether the marriage of Henry Fenwyk belonged to the king or not. The jurors stated that after the death of Henry's grandmother Elizabeth in 1410, Henry IV granted his marriage rights to William Folbery, who sold them to Henry's own mother Margaret, who sold them to Sir William Legh. Legh arranged Henry Fenwyk's marriage to his daughter Joan.[25] In February 1383, Richard II told Thomas Mowbray, the teenage heir to the earldom of Nottingham, that he could hold all his own lands currently in the king's hands if he married Elizabeth Lestrange (b. December 1373), heir to her late father Lord Lestrange of Blackmere. Nine-year-old Elizabeth, however, died in August 1383, and in 1384 Mowbray married the Earl of Arundel's daughter, also Elizabeth, without the king's permission. Richard II finally pardoned him in 1389.[26]

Seventeen-year-old Gilbert de Clare, Earl of Gloucester, sent envoys to Ireland to look at the four unmarried daughters of Richard de Burgh, Earl of Ulster (d. 1326), and they chose Maud as 'the fairest' of them. Gilbert married her in September 1308.[27] Thomas Longevilers of Nottinghamshire, aged twenty-one, was still unmarried in June 1300. The treasurer of England testified that 'the king [Edward I] had offered him one of the daughters of Adam Cretingges, deceased, and the heir having seen them agreed to marry the eldest'. Thomas had a much older sister, Ellota Longevilers, who had been set to marry twenty-three-year-old Henry Sutton on the Tuesday before Easter in 1279; Ellota's and Thomas's father, and Henry's uncle, had agreed that the couple would wed on that date. The two men, however, were unable to come to a final agreement regarding the marriage, and Henry wed a woman named Isabel the following February instead.[28] In October 1313, William Latimer, who owned the marriage rights of Hugh Poyntz (b. c. 1295), offered Hugh the hand of Joan Latimer, probably his niece.[29] Edward I granted the marriage rights of John Derle or d'Erleye, born in Derbyshire in February 1287, to Ralph Coterel, and Ralph offered John his daughter Maud. John 'affianced himself' to Maud Coterel, but in 1308 stated that in fact he had previously affianced himself to Letice Clifton, 'whom it was considered he would be compelled by ecclesiastical censure to marry'. By 1310, however, John was married to Maud Coterel after all.[30]

The whole system was extraordinarily unromantic, and provides an example of how, at the lower levels of society, people often had more freedom; they could at least choose their own spouse, and did not have to pay a massive fine for failing to marry the 'suitable' person offered to them. There is, however, evidence that marriages were still often arranged. On 9 February 1389, Thomas Sampson of Suffolk and John Otteleye of London made an indenture for the marriage of Thomas's son Simon Sampson and John's ward Margaret Knightcote, an orphan. Margaret had inherited 500 marks (£333.33) from her father William, a draper, and her guardian John Otteleye paid it to Thomas Sampson: £100 was in cash, and Sampson was to use the rest to purchase property for the couple and any children they might have, either together or if the survivor subsequently married a second spouse. Margaret and Simon were still married in the fifth year of Henry IV's reign (September 1403 to September 1404).[31] In October 1391, John Ourde rode almost forty miles from Harbottle, Northumberland to Newcastle-upon-Tyne to arrange his daughter Katherine's marriage. Two years earlier in Wimborne Minster, Dorset, twenty-eight-year-old Robert Syfryan met Edmund Brit in their parish church one Thursday in late October to arrange Robert's marriage to Edmund's daughter Christine. As 'they could not conclude owing to her absence', they decided to meet again three days later with Christine present. It is gratifying to note that a woman was able to consent to her own marriage and to take an active role in arranging it. In 1311, however, William Pervile and William Morton of Essex agreed between themselves that Pervile's sister Helen should marry Morton, and her own feelings on the matter were not recorded.[32]

Rank

Most people, whatever their station in life, married a partner of similar rank to themselves, and, often, who worked in a similar profession. Geoffrey Chaucer's *Miller's Tale* states *Man sholde wedde his simylitude* (Man should wed his equal) and *Men sholde wedden after hire estaat/ For youthe and elde is often at debaat* (Men should wed according to their station in life, for youth and old age are often in conflict). Kings often married kings' daughters, or failing that, the daughter of a duke or count. Richard II made a grand match in January 1382 when, just past his fifteenth birthday, he married Anne of Bohemia, eight months his senior and the daughter of the late Holy Roman Emperor, Charles IV. Having married an emperor's daughter, and realising as a widower in 1395/96 that he would have to marry again, Richard stated that he would only accept

Marriage (2)

a king's daughter as his second wife. This necessarily limited his options severely: the choices were either Yolande of Aragon (b. 1384), daughter of Juan II, King of Aragon (r. 1387–96), or one of the extremely young daughters of Charles VI, King of France (r. 1380–1422). Charles and his wife Isabeau of Bavaria were slightly younger than Richard himself, and their eldest daughter Isabelle de Valois was not quite seven when she married the twenty-nine-year-old king of England in late 1396. Richard was deposed by his cousin Henry IV less than three years later, and the marriage was never consummated.

Joan, illegitimate daughter of the London woolmonger John Ashford (d. 1329), married the London haberdasher John Levynge in 1335.[33] Rohese Romeyn (c. 1286–1329) was the eldest of the four daughters of Thomas Romeyn, mayor of London and a pepperer (i.e. an importer and seller of spices). Rohese's maternal uncle Philip Hauteyn was also a pepperer, and she married John Burford (d. 1322), another pepperer. John Preston, whose father of the same name was mayor of London in 1332/33, married Rohese Oxenford, whose father John Oxenford was mayor in 1341/42. Andrew Aubrey (d. 1358), was mayor of London from 1339 to 1341, and his son John (d. 1381) married Maud Fraunceys, granddaughter of Adam Fraunceys, mayor of London 1352/53. Maud's sister Agnes married William Staundon, mayor of London in 1392/93 and 1407/08. Maud herself, widowed from John Aubrey and her second husband Sir Alan Buxhill, constable of the Tower of London, made a brilliant third marriage when she wed John Montacute, Earl of Salisbury (d. 1400).

John of Gaunt, Duke of Lancaster (1340–99), son of Edward III, uncle of Richard II and father of Henry IV, married firstly Blanche of Lancaster, who was partly royal and was the enormously wealthy heir of the father the first Duke of Lancaster; secondly Constanza, daughter and heir of Pedro, King of Castile and Leon; and thirdly Katherine Swynford, née Roet, daughter of a herald, and widow of the Lincolnshire knight Sir Hugh Swynford. The marriage in 1396 of the woman who was the Duke of Lancaster's long-term lover and the mother of four of his children (the Beauforts, born in the 1370s) provides probably the most famous example of 'marrying up' in medieval England. Katherine Swynford's nephew Thomas Chaucer (*c.* 1367–1434), son of Katherine's sister Philippa and the great poet Geoffrey Chaucer, married the Oxfordshire heiress Maud Burghersh, probably as a result of Katherine's closeness to the powerful Duke of Lancaster. Thomas and Maud's daughter and heir Alice Chaucer (1404-75) became Countess of Salisbury by her second marriage and Duchess of Suffolk by her third, which, given that the Chaucers were a family of London merchants, is another remarkable example of marrying up.

It was not uncommon for a medieval noblewoman, having made an appropriate first marriage to a man of similar rank, to marry a second husband of lower standing. Edward I's daughter Joan of Acre (1272–1307) married firstly the wealthy and powerful Gilbert 'the Red' de Clare, Earl of Gloucester and Hertford, one of the greatest English noblemen of the late thirteenth century. A year after his death in late 1295, she secretly wed Gilbert's squire Ralph Monthermer. Her furious father confiscated her lands and imprisoned Monthermer when he heard of their marriage, though Joan defended her choice by stating 'It is not ignominious or shameful for a great and powerful earl to marry a poor woman of low rank. So, it is neither reprehensible nor problematic if a countess promotes a young strong man.'[34] Elizabeth Fitzalan (d. 1425), daughter of the Earl of Arundel, married firstly the Earl of Salisbury's son and heir, who was killed jousting in 1382 when they were both very young and childless, and secondly Thomas Mowbray, Earl of Nottingham and later Duke of Norfolk (d. September 1399). Sometime before 19 August 1401, Elizabeth married Robert Gousell, a squire who had worked for her second husband, in what was – given that she was a duchess and he was not even a knight – clearly a love match. Elizabeth and Robert's daughters were aged two and one in October 1403, so Elizabeth was probably already pregnant when they wed, and they had to acknowledge liability for a fine of 2,000 marks for marrying without Henry IV's permission. Elizabeth's lands were confiscated, though only for seven weeks.[35] Agnes Mortimer (d. 1368), daughter of the Earl of March and widow of the Earl of Pembroke (d. 1348), married secondly the obscure John Hakelut, who was not a knight, and Elizabeth Despenser (d. 1389), a great-granddaughter of Edward I, married Sir Maurice Wyth, a humble knight of the shire from Somerset, after the death of her first husband Lord Berkeley in 1368.[36]

Humphrey de Bohun, Earl of Hereford (1208–75) married firstly Mathilde de Lusignan, daughter of the French Count of Eu, and secondly Maud Avenbury, an Englishwoman of uncertain parentage. The brothers Thomas of Brotherton, Earl of Norfolk (1300–38) and Edmund of

Woodstock, Earl of Kent (1301–30) both married and had children with women further down the social scale than one would expect for men who were sons of a king of England (Edward I) and grandsons of a king of France (Philip III). Thomas's first wife was Alice Hales, whose father Roger was the coroner of Norfolk; his second was Mary Braose of the well-known Braose family, though only from a cadet branch. In 1325, Edmund married Margaret Wake, daughter of John, Lord Wake. Although Margaret came from a baronial family, her father was not an earl, and as she had two brothers, she was not an heiress. Edward II had attempted to arrange more fitting marriages for his half-brothers, with a daughter of the king of Aragon for Thomas and the daughter and heir of the French Viscount of Lomagne for Edmund, but when these matches fell through, the men took matters into their own hands.

Chapter 4

Marriage (3)

Second Marriages

Geoffroi de Charny stated in his *Book of Chivalry* that there were three possible ways of entering into marriage. Some men and women married when they had no carnal knowledge of the opposite sex, and married more for love (or lust) than riches; Geoffroi deemed this kind of marriage good, as it saved a couple from sin and provided heirs. The second kind was when an individual had no regard for the person s/he married, but did so out of greed for riches, and Charny believed 'it is unlikely that any good will come of it, for indeed the devils must be at their wedding'. The third kind was the marriage of those who were widowed, or old, or already had children with a previous spouse, and it was these people 'who live joyfully and pleasantly' in marriage, Charny claimed, more so than others.[1]

Second, and sometimes third, marriages were incredibly common, for both men and women; medieval England had no cultural expectation, as some societies did and do, that a widow should remain a widow and mourn for her husband for the rest of her life. Usually, it was considered respectful to wait a few months between the death of one's spouse and one's subsequent re-marriage, though not everyone abided by that unwritten rule. Juliana Leybourne, heir of her grandfather Lord Leybourne and a great landowner in Kent, married her third husband, Sir William Clinton, later Earl of Huntingdon, within two months of her second husband Sir Thomas Blount's death in 1328. Her first husband, John, Lord Hastings, had died in January 1325, and she received royal permission to marry Blount in July that year.[2] The Earl of Derby's daughter Eleanor Ferrers (d. 1274) lost her first husband William Vaux shortly before 14 September 1252, and married Roger Quency, Earl of Winchester, before 5 December 1252, without a royal licence.[3] Robert Convers, a goldsmith, died shortly before 27 July 1310, leaving his

Marriage (3)

children Nicholas, Henry and Katherine, aged seven, three and one respectively. His widow Rohese married David Cottesbroke very soon afterwards, before 29 August 1310, and thirdly Nicholas Stratstede before June 1321.[4] Katherine, widow of Nicholas Crane, alderman of London, also remarried quickly after her husband's death. Nicholas made his will on 15 April 1342 and it was proved on 27 May; Katherine was married to Nicholas Poure of Bletchingdon, Oxfordshire by 17 August 1342.[5]

Blanche Mowbray (c. late 1330s–1409), daughter of Lord Mowbray (1310–68) and granddaughter of the royal Earl of Lancaster and Leicester, was married five times, though had no surviving children. Her parents arranged a marriage for her on 13 March 1342 to Edward Montacute, nephew of the Earl of Salisbury and a great-grandson of Edward I, and the wedding was to take place around 24 June 1343. They were both small children at the time. Edward Montacute was alive in June 1349 but dead by December 1359, and it may be that their marriage was never consummated.[6] Blanche's second husband Robert Bertram, Baron of Bothal in Northumberland, died in 1363, and she married her third, Thomas, Lord Poynings, in 1372. Born in 1349, Thomas was about a decade her junior, and died in his mid-twenties; in his will, he called his wife by her maiden name, 'Blanch de Mowbray'. Blanche married her fourth husband, John Worth (d. 1391), in 1377, and her fifth and last, John Wiltshire, in 1394.[7] Elizabeth Fitzalan married four husbands: after she was widowed from Robert Gousell (see above) in 1403, she wed Sir Gerard Usflete. Katherine Neville (late 1390s–1483), daughter of the Earl of Westmorland and a great-granddaughter of Edward III, was also married four times, firstly to John Mowbray, Duke of Norfolk (d. 1432), and subsequently to Lord Strangeways (d. 1442/43) and Lord Beaumont (d. 1460). Beaumont was born in 1409 and was about ten years her junior. Katherine's fourth marriage to Queen Elizabeth Woodville's brother Sir John Woodville in early 1465 was slammed by contemporaries as 'diabolical'; he was close to fifty years younger than she. Remarkably, however, Katherine outlived him.

Second and third marriages meant that a lot of people had stepchildren and stepparents, and were often close to them. Philip Bret, who made his will in July 1316, left tenements and shops in London to his own children Laurence and Christine, and 'a solar with a fireplace' to Isabel, daughter of his late wife Maud from her previous marriage. The will of Henry Chaundeler was proved in February 1317, and he left his stepson

Maurice, his wife Isabel's son, his shop and 100s worth of candles. Richard Kyng, a butcher, left money to his own daughters Emma and Isabel and to his stepdaughter Millecent, his deceased first wife Joan's daughter, in 1347, and in 1348 Roger Forsham, mercer and sheriff of London, who had no children of his own, left bequests to his wife Alice's daughters Maud and Christine, his sister Lucy's daughters Agnes and Cecile, and his sister Margaret's daughter Agnes.[8]

Marriages and second marriages among the nobility sometimes created almost impossible tangles. William Ferrers, Earl of Derby (d. 1254), married firstly Sybil Marshal, daughter of the Earl of Pembroke, and secondly Margaret Quency, daughter of Roger Quency, Earl of Winchester. Eleanor Ferrers, one of William and Sybil's seven daughters, married Roger Quency, and thus became the stepmother of her stepmother. For William Ferrers and Margaret Quency's five children, this meant that their half-sister married their grandfather, and it is perhaps just as well that Eleanor and Roger had no children. Edward I's daughter Joan of Acre had four children from her first marriage to Gilbert de Clare, who had two daughters from his own first marriage to Alice de Lusignan and was already a grandfather to Duncan MacDuff, future Earl of Fife, when he wed eighteen-year-old Joan in 1290. Joan had another four children from her second marriage to Ralph Monthermer, and their daughter Mary Monthermer (1297–c. 1371) married Duncan MacDuff, grandson of her mother's first husband. Joan and Gilbert's four de Clare children saw their half-sister marry their half-nephew. Gwladus Ddu, also known as Gwladys ferch Llywelyn (d. 1251), married firstly Reginald Braose (d. 1228), Lord of Brecon and Abergavenny, and secondly Ralph Mortimer (d. 1246), Lord of Wigmore. Gwladus and Ralph's son Roger Mortimer (b. early 1230s) married Maud Braose, granddaughter of Reginald Braose from his first marriage, and thus Gwladus's step-granddaughter. Maud's father was William Braose, whom Gwladus Ddu's father Llywelyn Fawr, Prince of Gwynedd, hanged in 1230 for committing adultery with Llywelyn's English wife Joan, almost certainly Gwladus's mother. The sisters Eleanor (c. 1366–99) and Mary (c. 1370–94) de Bohun, joint heirs to the earldoms of Hereford, Essex and Northampton, married an uncle and nephew: Thomas of Woodstock, Edward III's youngest son, and Henry of Lancaster, Edward III's grandson. And finally, in c. 1371 Sir Peter Mauley and his son from his first marriage, also Peter Mauley, married two sisters, Constance and Margery Sutton.

Marriage (3)

Dowry

The medieval bride was expected to provide a dowry on marriage, and not only at the highest levels of society. Many merchants and tradesmen bequeathed sums of money in their wills to daughters, sisters or nieces 'for their marriage'. The sums varied according to the wealth of the individual: Joce Evatte, a clerk, left six marks (960d) for his daughter Agnes's marriage in 1363, whereas three years later, Adam Brabason was able to leave £50 (12,000d) as his daughter Joan's marriage portion. Richard Wycombe gave his six-year-old daughter Isabel 200 marks of silver for her future dowry in 1358, and in 1390, William Tonge left each of his daughters 100 marks (16,000d) as marriage portions, 'which sum is to be reduced to 100s (1,200d) should they marry without discretion or live immodestly'. When Alice Samford married Stephen Goding in Essex on 21 October 1286, her brother Richard gave Stephen twenty marks (3,200d) as her dowry.[9]

Some well-off men willed money so that 'poor girls' would be able to marry. John Longe, a vintner, left bequests 'for marriage portions for poor girls throughout the city of London' in his will of 1361. Thomas Mockyng, who was a clerk on low pay but came from a family of well-off fishmongers, requested in 1428 that the residue of his estate be used to provide 'poor maidens' marriage portions'. Sometimes money or property was willed to a daughter not yet born for her future marriage: when he made his will in or before April 1361, John Ryvel suspected that his wife Joan was pregnant, and left her their London house. If the unborn child was a boy, he would inherit the house after Joan's death; if a girl, the house was to be sold to provide her dowry. When John Doget and Idonea Birlyngham married in July 1385, John's father Walter and Idonea's stepfather John Philipot each gave the couple £100. Idonea had also been left £100 by her late father John Birlyngham for her dowry.[10]

Wealthy noblemen were, of course, able to provide much greater dowries for their daughters. In the late 1250s, Philip, Lord Basset (d. 1271) gave the Northamptonshire manor of Barnwell to his daughter and heir Aline when she married Sir Hugh Despenser, and William Beauchamp (d. 1298), Earl of Warwick, gave the villages of Hartley Mauditt in Hampshire and Chedworth in Gloucestershire to his daughter Isabella when she married her first husband Patrick Chaworth around 1280. By 1348, Sir Robert Corbet, previously 'rich and powerful', had brought himself to penury by his 'great liberality' in providing dowries for his daughters.[11] Twelve-year-old Richard II came close to marrying Caterina Visconti, daughter of the exceedingly rich Lord of Milan and Pavia, in 1379, though ultimately he married Anne of Bohemia, daughter of the late Holy Roman Emperor. Chroniclers grumbled that Anne brought prestigious family connections but no dowry, whereas if Richard had married into the Viscontis they would have given him, and England, a fabulous sum of money.

Dower and the Courtesy of England

Usually, an Englishwoman who married a man who owned lands and property and died before her had the legal right to hold one-third of his lands as dower for the rest of her life. In London, the custom was different: 'a widow took a third part if there were children, and one half if there were no children'.[12] Otherwise, the right to hold a third of one's late husband's or husbands' estate applied regardless of whether the couple had children, or whether the widow married again, or how wealthy she was in her own right. As noted above, the 'courtesy of England' gave a man who married an heiress the right to keep all her lands for the rest of his own life if she died before him, but only if they had a child together; if not, on her death her lands passed to her heir by blood. In 1281, Roger Bigod, Earl of Norfolk (c. 1245–1306), claimed that his recently deceased wife Aline Basset, heir of the wealthy Basset family, had borne him a child in Woking, Surrey who took a breath before dying. Aline's twenty-year-old son and heir from her first marriage, Hugh Despenser, vigorously challenged his stepfather, who abandoned the claim; Aline's lands passed intact to Hugh.[13]

John of Gaunt, Duke of Lancaster, was one of the greatest beneficiaries of the 'courtesy of England' in the Middle Ages. In 1359, he married Blanche of Lancaster, younger daughter and one of the two co-heirs of Henry of Grosmont, first Duke of Lancaster and Earl of Derby, Leicester and Lincoln. When Blanche's older sister Maud died childless in her early twenties in 1362, Blanche came into the entire Lancastrian inheritance, with lands and castles in thirty-four English counties and across Wales. She died at the age of twenty-six in 1368, and as she and John had children together, he had the right to hold all her enormous inheritance for the remaining thirty years of his life. It made him one of the richest men in medieval England, with an annual gross income of about £12,000.

A statute passed in 1285 held that a woman who deserted her husband and was not reconciled to him at the time of his death forfeited her right to dower. Margaret Gatesden, who left her husband John Camoys in or before 1277 and lived with her lover William Paynel, had to fight for her rightful Camoys dower after John died in 1298 (see also Chapter 6 below). Another case was Alice, wife of Jordan Bacheler of Surrey (d. 1297), who was accused of leaving her husband and living in adultery, and 'was not reconciled to the said Jordan before his death, so that she ought not to have her dower'. An inquisition found, however, that Jordan had taken a mistress named Maud Tayllour, and 'behaved so ill towards Alice his wife that she could not live with him; thus she did not leave her husband nor desert him with evil intent or in adultery, but to avoid danger to herself, she betook herself from him to her parents', where she lived 'virtuously' and committed no adultery. She was therefore granted her rightful dower.[14]

Chapter 5

Marriage (4)

Abductions and Forced Marriages

Although noblewomen, especially those who owned lands, were in some ways more protected and respected than women of lower rank, they faced a particular danger: abduction. There is little doubt that when a woman was abducted and forcibly married, the consummation of the marriage she had not agreed to or wished for was rape.

Margaret Audley, heir to a third of her late uncle Gilbert de Clare's earldom of Gloucester, was only about fourteen when she was abducted from her parents' home in Thaxted, Essex in early 1336.[1] Her kidnapper was Sir Ralph Stafford, a widower twenty years her senior, who was aided in his unlawful endeavour by a large number of his relatives and adherents (eighteen named men and unnamed, uncounted 'others'). Margaret was forced to marry Ralph, and ultimately bore him two sons and four daughters before her death in 1349. Ralph Stafford was a friend of Edward III and suffered no punishment whatsoever as a result of his abduction and rape of a noblewoman who was the king's cousin. Not only was Ralph never punished, he thrived: he made himself and his descendants the owners of Margaret Audley's large inheritance, became the first Earl of Stafford in 1351, and lived until 1372 when he was over seventy. His and Margaret's Stafford descendants became dukes of Buckingham in the early fifteenth century, and were some of the most prominent people in England during the Wars of the Roses and the early Tudor era. This all came about because of Ralph's abduction of Margaret Audley; before 1336, the Staffords held only a few manors in the Midlands and were insignificant compared to their later wealth and prominence.[2] Margaret's aunts Elizabeth de Burgh and Eleanor Despenser, sisters of the Earl of Gloucester and his other co-heirs, were also abducted and forcibly married, in 1316 and in 1329 as widows of

Marriage (4)

twenty and thirty-six respectively. The massive de Clare estate proved something of a poisoned chalice for the women who inherited it.

Maud Clifford was the daughter and heir of Walter Clifford (d. 1263) and Marared ferch Llywelyn, and married William Longespee, Earl of Salisbury (d. 1256/57), with whom she had one child, Margaret, Countess of Salisbury and Lincoln. On 1 October 1270, fourteen years after she was widowed, Maud was forcibly taken from her manor of Canford in Dorset by John, Lord Giffard of Brimpsfield, and a 'great multitude of armed men'. The abduction came to Henry III's ears four days later on 5 October, and he demonstrated concern for Maud's wellbeing and ordered Giffard to appear before him and explain himself on pain of forfeiting all his lands. Giffard duly appeared and claimed that he did not abduct Maud against her will, but the statement that on 10 March 1271 she was 'so inflicted by infirmity that she cannot come before the king at present' is surely revealing.[3] Katherine, the eldest of John Giffard and Maud Clifford's three daughters, appears to have been born in 1272, and one might speculate that Maud became pregnant as a result of rape and therefore came to the conclusion that she had little choice but to marry her abductor and rapist.[4]

Maud Clifford's granddaughter Alice de Lacy (1281–1348), Countess of Lincoln in her own right and the Lacy and Longespee heir, married Edward I's nephew Thomas of Lancaster (d. 1322) in 1294. Alice left Thomas in 1317 with the aid of the Earl of Surrey, John de Warenne, and fled from Thomas while staying at Canford in Dorset, which she inherited from her mother and grandmother. This rather curious and unusual situation appears to have been a voluntary act on Alice's part, rather than an abduction as claimed by several contemporary chroniclers. The widowed Alice married Sir Eble Lestrange in 1324, much more happily and willingly. Mere weeks after Eble died in September 1335, Sir Hugh Frene abducted the now fifty-four-year-old Alice from her own home of Bolingbroke Castle in Lincolnshire, and forcibly married her. Frene was only briefly imprisoned by Edward III for doing so. A petition Alice sent to the king makes her distress, anger and humiliation all too painfully apparent, and to make matters even worse, her own half-brother John had aided Frene's abduction of her. Alice's only comfort was that Hugh Frene died fighting in Scotland barely a year later, and she outlived him by a dozen years.[5]

Alice Newby of Skipton-on-Swale in Yorkshire was abducted by Thomas Peron in August 1413. Peron, his two brothers and eleven other men rode to the field near Skipton where Alice was haying with her mother and brothers, and carried her off. They soon encountered another group of men on horseback, who became suspicious and questioned Alice if all was well. According to the later testimony of this group's leader, William Berkesworth, Alice stated that it was her parents' will that she and Thomas Peron should marry, and the two of them took their marriage vows there and then, on horseback. What happened next is unclear but apparently, Berkesworth decided to take Alice back to her parents, perhaps realising despite her protestations that she was not there of her own accord, and her parents subsequently kept her away from Thomas Peron. Thomas sued Alice, claiming that they had legally contracted marriage; she claimed that her consent had been forced. The case was resolved in Alice's favour.[6] Another fifteenth-century example of abduction is Jane Wichingham, one of the daughters and heirs of Edmund Wichingham, taken from her parents' home in Wood Rising, Norfolk by Robert Langstrother and up to sixty armed men in June 1451.[7]

Being an heiress carried heavy risks for girls and women, and not only for wealthy noblewomen. Shortly before April 1378, eleven-year-old Joan Hampstede, heir of her late maternal grandfather, was abducted from her home and from her father Walter's care by Joan Wodelok and Ralph Taillour. When she came of age, Joan Hampstede was set to inherit a house, forty acres of land and ten acres of wood in the village of South Mimms in Middlesex.[8] Joan Wodelok and Ralph Taillour's objective in abducting the child was not stated, but they surely intended to marry her to Joan Wodelok's son; Taillour claimed to the authorities that Joan had 'procured' him to aid and abet her felony. Isabel Wycombe was born in early 1352 to a well-off London rope-maker, Richard Wycombe, and his second wife Pernel. Richard left Isabel 200 marks of silver as her dowry and his 'best silver *spicedisshe*' in his will, and the temptation of such a large marriage portion proved too great for someone: within weeks of her father's death in 1361, nine-year-old Isabel was 'carried off and could not be found'. Horribly, it transpired during an investigation seven years later that the child had died not long after her abduction.[9]

Unfortunately for women and girls, abduction usually paid off for the men who took them from their homes, and forcibly married them; there were massive benefits and few risks – a fine and temporary imprisonment at worst – for the abductors. Once a couple was married, only the pope could unmarry them, and without a pre-existing impediment, he could not and would not do so. A woman's or girl's lack of consent, her kidnapping from her home or her parents' home, and her ordeal of experiencing what certainly amounted to rape, did not count as impediments.

Thomas Norwich, a chaplain, was questioned in July 1382 on the grounds that he had broken into Henry Wilton's home on several occasions and had 'carried away the plaintiff's wife Joan, woollen and linen cloths, silver plate, dishes, pewter salt-cellars and iron and brass and pots and pans'. Not only was the unfortunate Joan added to this list as though she were merely another piece of her husband's tableware, a jury brought in the verdict that 'as regards the wife, she was nothing but a common strumpet' and that therefore there was no forced abduction. If a woman could be deemed a 'common strumpet', abducting her was no felony, it seems. A similar case had been heard a few months earlier in September 1381: Richard Elme, baker of London, accused the fishmonger John Hankyn of abducting and carrying away his wife Alice, as well as his woollen cloths, four cups with silver bands, two pieces of silver and eight gold rings.[10] Although on this occasion Alice Elme was not accused of being a 'common strumpet', she was, like Joan Wilton, lumped together with her husband's stolen possessions.

Some boys were also victims of abduction and forced marriage. William Huberd, a minter of London, died in March or April 1328, and custody of his ten-year-old son Robert was given to John Spray. On 20 November 1331, Robert Huberd, now thirteen, was abducted from his guardian's home by William Rameseye, his wife Christine, his father William the elder and a few others including the chaplain of Woolchurch-Haw, and was forcibly married to William and Christine's daughter Agnes. The Rameseyes appeared before the court of the mayor of London a few days later, and 'inasmuch as the marriage could not be annulled', Robert Huberd was given the choice of remaining with his in-laws or returning to his guardian. He chose the Rameseyes.[11]

In 1315, a boy or young man named Thomas Fraunceys, son and heir of the late Adam Fraunceys, was abducted from his mother Joan's custody in Beckingham, Yorkshire. In the same year, also in Yorkshire, John Lilling, son and heir of the late Simon, was abducted from his guardian's house, and in 1316 John Comberton, son and heir of the late Philip, was abducted from the Cambridge home of his guardians Roger and Margery Peyntour. One of John's abductors was Joan Comberton, his nearest living relative.[12] In or soon before March 1337, Reynold

Rokesle's widow Joan abducted Reynold's eight-year-old nephew and heir Richard Rokesle, and detained him in St Mary Cray, a manor she had held jointly with Reynold.[13] Ten- or twelve-year-old John Chaucer, later the father of the poet Geoffrey (born c. 1342), was abducted in 1324 by his aunt Agnes, who hoped to marry him to her daughter and thereby keep property in Ipswich within the family. The royal writs ordering the arrest and imprisonment of Agnes and her husband call this abduction 'ravishing'.[14] In c. 1308/09, four men abducted the underage Henry Frowyk from his mother Agnes's custody, took him to the Earl of Hereford's castle of Pleshey in Essex, and married him (to an unnamed wife) against Agnes's will.[15]

In all these cases, the motive for abduction was an attempt to benefit financially from the custody of an heir and his/her marriage, which could be valuable. It was not, however, without risks. The Second Statute of Westminster in 1285 set the punishment for abducting a child (whether male or female) whose marriage belonged to someone else at two years' imprisonment, as long as the person restored the child still unmarried, or paid what the marriage was worth. Otherwise, the punishment was either life imprisonment or abjuration of the realm, i.e. permanent exile from England.[16] Although boys and young men were sometimes abducted and forcibly married, once they came of age at twenty-one, this danger passed; this was not the case for women, who could be and sometimes were abducted at any age.

One abduction had a rather happier ending. Maud Clifford (b. 1270s), widow of Robert, Lord Clifford (1274–1314), was abducted by John the Irishman in early November 1315, and taken to Barnard Castle in County Durham. A few days later, Edward II sent a contingent of knights and men-at-arms to rescue Lady Clifford, and one of the knights was Sir Robert Welle. Romantically, Maud married Sir Robert shortly after he and his associates rescued her from John the Irishman's clutches, though less romantically, the king confiscated her lands and goods for marrying Robert without his permission.[17]

Disputed and Unhappy Marriages

John Giffard of Brimpsfield, the man who abducted Maud Clifford in 1270, was born c. 1232/33 as the son and heir of Sir Elias Giffard (d. 1248). John was four years old when he was contracted to marry

Aubrey Camville, who was about four or five, and as noted above, they married in 1241 when they were both about eight, and Aubrey was taller than John. A juror many years later said, however, that 'he often heard the said John declaiming against the marriage ... and never saw them together after they were 12 or 14 years old, nor did he ever exhibit her in any of his manors'. Another juror said that he also often heard the said John declaiming against his marriage, and heard him say that 'no-one of the race of Longespey [a noble family] would adhere to any wife to whom he happened to be married in his boyhood ... but he knows not whether this was said in joke'. A third man said that he 'heard him declaim against the marriage ... the said Aubrey stayed at the said John's manor ... and she asked him why he ... [*words missing*] he answered nothing but afterwards always avoided her presence'.[18]

Annulment of a marriage was extremely difficult and could in any case only be done by the pope, and in most cases, incompatible couples had little choice but to remain married. Marriage meant for life, almost without exception. Edmund, Earl of Cornwall (b. 1249) was a nephew of Henry III, and married the Earl of Gloucester's sister Margaret de Clare in 1272. Margaret was pregnant in early 1285, but either she lost the infant or it died in infancy, and marital relations deteriorated. By 1289, Pope Nicholas IV and John Peckham, Archbishop of Canterbury, had intervened, and Peckham excommunicated Edmund for his refusal to cohabit with Margaret. The couple officially separated in 1294, and Edmund settled £800 of land annually on his estranged wife. For her part, Margaret, whether willingly or not, took a vow of chastity as long as Edmund was alive (he died in 1300 and she outlived him by a dozen years).[19]

Margaret Marshal (c. 1322–99), Countess and later Duchess of Norfolk in her own right, was the elder daughter and ultimately the sole heir of Edward I's son Thomas of Brotherton, Earl of Norfolk and Earl Marshal of England. She was unhappily married to John, Lord Segrave (b. 1315), with whom she had one surviving child, Elizabeth, Lady Mowbray (b. 1338). The date of Margaret and John's wedding is not recorded, but John's marriage was granted to Margaret's father Thomas in March 1327 when Margaret was about four or five. In 1350/51, Margaret tried to have her marriage annulled on the grounds that she was 'contracted to him before she was of marriageable age, and has never agreed to cohabit with him'. The 'matrimonial cause' between Margaret and John was to be tried before the Dean of Poitiers, a papal auditor, and the Bishop of London. Ultimately, the marriage was never annulled, but Segrave died in April 1353 anyway, and the following year Margaret married her second husband, Sir Walter Manny, without her cousin Edward III's permission. The king imprisoned her 'honourably' in Somerton Castle in Lincolnshire in July 1354, with her servants and with conjugal visits allowed, and pardoned the couple in December 1355.[20]

The case of Richard Fitzalan and Isabella Despenser was similar. Richard, the seven-year-old son and heir of the Earl of Arundel, was married to Isabella, eight-year-old eldest daughter of the Lord of Glamorgan and a great-granddaughter of Edward I, in February 1321. In December 1344, Richard complained to the pope that he and Isabella had been married as children before they could consent, and were 'forced by blows to cohabit' when they reached puberty (who hit them to make them sleep together, assuming the story was true, was not explained). Mere weeks later, Richard married his second wife Eleanor of Lancaster, widow of Lord Beaumont and daughter of the Earl of Lancaster, and his and Isabella's teenage son Edmund was made illegitimate by the annulment. Deceit was involved in Richard and Eleanor's marriage: firstly they claimed that they did not know they were third cousins, which, given that they were both members of the tiny English noble elite, is all but impossible. Secondly, they concealed Eleanor's true identity from the pope until after they were safely married by calling her 'Joan Beaumont' and by claiming that she was related to Isabella Despenser via her father, when in fact she was Isabella's cousin via her mother.[21]

Margaret Pressen was married to John Lutre in the 1340s when he was nine and she was also underage, and she had the marriage annulled when she came of age 'for want of consent' and married Thomas Gray in c. 1352 instead.[22] Mary Percy (1368–94) was the only child of Henry, Lord Percy (c. 1321–68) and his second wife Joan Oreby (c. 1351–69), and was the heir of the Oreby family. Mary was married as a child in early 1377 to John Southeray (b. c. early 1360s), illegitimate son of Edward III and his mistress Alice Perrers. After King Edward died a few months later, Mary and her much older half-brother Henry Percy, Earl of Northumberland, managed to have her marriage annulled on the grounds that John was too 'plebeian' to be her husband. She subsequently married John, Lord Ros, a grandson of the Earl of Stafford.[23]

Pope Sixtus IV dealt with the case of Margery Platte of the diocese of Coventry and Lichfield in 1476. She stated that 'when under age and constrained by fear', she was forced to marry Thurstan Platte, and when she came of age she repudiated the marriage and asked John Hales, Bishop of Coventry and Lichfield, to annul the marriage. Thurstan, however, claimed that Margery had committed 'adultery and fornication' with Sir John Trafford, and Bishop Hales excommunicated her. John Trafford protested that two men had deliberately provided false information, and Sixtus absolved him and Margery. In 1435, Pope Eugene IV accused Richard Brune of bringing about a divorce between James Hopwode and Joan Rikil of the diocese of Rochester by deception, because he wished to marry Joan himself and gain access to her large inheritance. Richard and Joan, who had left James and also wished to marry Richard, persuaded various witnesses to give false testimony regarding her marriage to James, and when an annulment was granted, she married Richard instead. Pope Eugene ordered Joan to return to James Hopwode and declared her second marriage invalid.[24]

In 1378, Margery Nerford (c. 1360–1417) of Norfolk, daughter and heir of John Nerford (d. 1363), petitioned the pope for an annulment of her marriage to John Brewes, and also petitioned the government of the child-king Richard II stating that she 'fears injury from the said John and his accomplices'. She was right to fear them: while Margery was staying in London with her grandmother, Alice Nevill, Brewes and his men broke in and abducted her, intending to prevent her from attempting to end the marriage. They took her to the Thames-side palace of the Bishop of Norwich, from where Brewes' adherent Sir Robert Howard took her to Chelsea and then 'carried her off from one county to another, keeping her in secret places'. Howard was caught and imprisoned in the Tower, though freed on condition that he made every effort to bring Margery before the royal council; he eventually did so, and Margery was restored to her grandmother. The annulment case dragged on into the 1380s but was eventually resolved in Margery's favour, and she took a vow of chastity. She died in 1417, and her former husband John in 1426, having married a second wife, Margaret Poynings.[25]

Impediments and Domestic Abuse

One impediment to a marriage that could cause it to be annulled was a spiritual connection between the couple that had received no dispensation (see 'Baptism and Godparents' in Chapter 9 for more information). It might have been permitted under English law for men to hit their wives, but women were not expected to tolerate excessive abuse. A victim of domestic violence could apply to the courts for a divorce (or rather, an annulment) *a mensa et thoro*, 'from bed and board', on the grounds of her husband's cruelty or adultery.[26] In York in 1345, Agnes Huntyngdon left her husband, Simon Munkton, a goldsmith. Munkton sought the assistance of the Archbishop of York, William Zouche (d. 1352), who charged Agnes with deserting her husband without just cause. Agnes alleged that she had left Simon because he beat her and she was frightened of him, and furthermore, that she had pre-contracted marriage with John of Bristol and therefore was not Simon's legal wife.[27] In 1300, an ecclesiastical court ordered Thomas Louchard of Droitwich in Worcestershire to be whipped for beating his wife with a stick, and in 1315 Emma Baker of Pilsgate (near Stamford in Lincolnshire) called for her brother John Reeve's help when her husband John Baker beat her. Reeve, 'with Emma's approval', took matters into his own hands by hitting Baker on the head with a hatchet, and killed him. The siblings were both arrested.[28]

Mabel Smith of London obtained a judicial separation from her husband Robert in 1457 on the grounds that he had 'shamelessly committed adultery' with numerous women and 'was treating her so cruelly that she could no longer cohabit with him without danger of her person', and Anne Cope of the diocese of Lincoln was granted a separation from her husband John in 1475, because he cheated on her with many women and 'behaved to her with such violence that it was not safe for her to live with him'. Cristina Sewale of London also obtained a judicial separation from her husband John Archer in 1457 because he 'has so inhumanly beaten and wounded her beyond her deserts, even when she was pregnant, that he caused her to bring forth two stillborn children, and still treats her so cruelly that she is in fear of her life'. Although it was far less common, men could also be granted an annulment if their wives were cruel and abusive or adulterous. John Marston petitioned the dean of London in 1400, stating that his wife Alice had committed adultery and he dared not live with her because she 'has, he knows not why, several times sought his death'.[29]

One exception to the rule that a pre-existing impediment or cruelty was required to annul a marriage was a man's impotence, and therefore, the non-consummation of the marriage. In July 1370, a vintner of

London, William Sharpyng, helped his wife Joan Coutenhale annul their marriage on the grounds of his impotence. William 'agreed to appear before a judge in court and submit to examination, so that it might appear whether he was impotent or not'. This examination might have followed the procedure laid out by the English theologian Thomas Chobham (d. 1230) in his *Summa Confessorum*: 'After food and drink, the man and woman are to be placed together in one bed and wise women are to be summoned around the bed for many nights. And if the man's member is always found useless as if dead, the couple are well able to be separated'. In or before 1429, Alice Russell of York requested an annulment of her marriage to John Skathelok because he was impotent. The female witnesses, perhaps prostitutes, who inspected John exposed their breasts and genitalia to him and attempted to arouse him with explicit language. Joan Gilbert complained of her husband John Marche's impotence in 1441, and three women, Joan Savage, Agnes Grey and Joan Rande, kissed and embraced John and touched his penis to test his impotence, though remained dressed and did not use explicit language.[30]

Richard Lyons died in London on 13 June 1381, during the Great Uprising or Peasants' Revolt, and his widow Isabella Pledour claimed half of his goods to the value of 1,500 marks, in accordance with the London custom that a widow could take half of her late husband's estate if they had no children and a third if they did. Richard's executors, however, stated that Richard and Isabella's marriage had been annulled in 1363 'on account of certain impediments'. Isabella admitted that this was true but appealed against the annulment, and the case dragged on until 1391. To complicate matters, it was said that Richard was 'a bastard who died without heir' and therefore his estate should have escheated to the Crown.[31] A famous case of a medieval annulment, or rather two annulments, is that of Jacqueline, Countess of Hainault (1401–36), whose third husband was Humphrey, Duke of Gloucester (1390–1447), brother of Henry V and uncle of Henry VI. Jacqueline was widowed from the Dauphin of France in April 1417 before she even turned sixteen, and married Jan IV, Duke of Brabant (b. 1403) in 1418; the teenage couple were soon estranged, and the marriage was annulled. Jacqueline secretly married Humphrey sometime in early 1423. In 1425, Pope Martin V declared that her marriage to Jan IV of Brabant had not been properly annulled and that therefore her marriage to Humphrey was illegitimate, and this marriage too was annulled in 1428. Jacqueline wed her fourth and last husband, Frank van Borssele, some years later.

Some couples who were unable to have their marriage annulled nevertheless lived apart. In London in 1305, Alice Frowyk lived alone, having separated from her husband Thomas.[32] The problem for women, however, was that, according to the Second Statute of Westminster, if they voluntarily left their husbands and lived with a lover, they had no rights to dower after the death of their husband unless he had forgiven them and they were reconciled at the time of his death.[33] Even if women did not commit adultery and wished to live alone, as Alice Frowyk did, it was extremely hard, given bars on women entering numerous professions and judgemental attitudes, for single women to earn their own living. Another issue was the Church's insistence that marriage was a sacrament and the Biblical directive 'what God hath joined together, let no man put asunder'. A woman who left her husband not only potentially made her living situation very precarious, but risked putting her soul in jeopardy. Some women were excommunicated for refusing to live with their husbands, such as Christine Verner in 1388, or were suspended, a lesser form of excommunication where a person was forbidden to take the Eucharist and the sacraments, such as Katherine Kyrton in 1463.[34] Alice Frowyk's husband Thomas came from a wealthy family of goldsmiths, and possibly the couple came to a financial arrangement which enabled Alice to live by herself, but this carried further risks: she was assaulted and robbed in her own home shortly before 15 December 1305 by a thief named Roger Rokesle and eighteen associates. They broke into Alice's home, assaulted her and threw her out into the street, and stole her gold and silver jewellery to a value of £40.[35]

Chapter 6

Sexual Pleasure and Relationships (1)

Sexual Pleasure and Desire

John Gaddesden, born c. 1280 and a graduate of the University of Oxford, is perhaps the most famous English physician of the later Middle Ages. In his *Rosa Anglica* ('English Rose'), Gaddesden wrote:

> To excite and arouse a woman to intercourse, a man ought to speak, kiss and embrace [her], to touch her breasts, to caress her breasts and to touch the whole [area] between her perineum and her vulva, and to strike her buttocks with the purpose that the woman desires sex [...] and when the woman begins to stammer, then they ought to copulate.[1]

In stark contrast to the opinions of later centuries, medieval England believed that women experienced more pleasure in intercourse than men, and that women's need for intercourse was insatiable and stronger than men's. Another common belief was that both men and women emitted seed that united to create an embryo, and it followed that if a woman felt a 'lack of pleasure' she did not emit this 'sperm' and therefore, no conception could take place. Medical belief in the Middle Ages, by holding that women must orgasm in order to conceive a child, followed Galen.[2] A further idea was that male seed was precious and should not be wasted, while female seed was both prodigious and potentially lethal unless frequently purged. Menstruation achieved this, as did intercourse, and masturbation was recommended to avoid the dangers of a woman storing up her 'seed'. If she did not, she would suffer from an affliction called 'uterine suffocation', which would cause her to have difficulty breathing and to endure fainting fits and convulsions. John Gaddesden stated:

> If the suffocation comes from a retention of the sperm, the woman should get together with and draw up a marriage contract with some man. If she does not or cannot do this, because she is a nun and it is forbidden by her monastic vow or because she is married to an old man incapable of giving her her due, she should travel overseas, take vigorous exercise and use medicine which will dry up the sperm ... if she has a fainting fit, the midwife should insert a finger covered with oil of lily, laurel or spikenard into her womb and move it vigorously about.[3]

The twelfth-century *Trotula* stated that women who were not permitted to have carnal intercourse, because they were nuns or widows or otherwise vowed to chastity, risked 'grave illness' if they wished to have intercourse and did not do so. As a remedy, such women were advised to anoint some cotton with pennyroyal oil and insert it in the vagina, or if they had no such oil, to dissolve trifera magna with a little warm wine and to place it in the vagina with cotton or damp wool. This, the authors confidently asserted, would cause the women's desire for intercourse to recede.[4]

In his 1354 treatise *The Book of Holy Medicines*, Henry of Grosmont, first Duke of Lancaster, wrote that a 'great deal of the sin of lechery enters through this gateway', meaning eyesight. He stated that 'when I have trapped some foolish woman with my smooth and beguiling words, it pleases me so much to look at her, and with such overwhelming lecherous pleasure, that for the time I think of nothing else. And it seems to me that I was so inflamed by the fire of lechery through that sin that whatever she did I loved above all else and I saw nothing I didn't like.' He added that he would rather 'kiss', which is a euphemism, 'an ugly, poor tramp' (*une lede poure garce* in the French original) than a good woman of high status, however lovely she was, and the more she loved and served God, the less it pleased him to kiss her. Henry admitted to dancing elegantly so that women would admire him, and added that although dancing itself was not sinful, his intentions were, because dancing caused him to commit the sin of lechery: it aroused in him the sinful desire to 'be admired, then loved, then lost'.[5]

Medieval women, it seems, enjoyed the sight of men's legs and arms. Duke Henry stated in his *Holy Medicines* that he stretched out his legs in his stirrups at jousting tournaments so that female spectators would admire his calves, and that in his youth he showed off and was proud of his strong arms, shapely hands and the rings on his fingers.[6] Geoffrey Chaucer's Wife of Bath, whose given name was Alisoun, fell in lust with her much younger fifth husband Jankyn at her fourth husband's funeral, while Jankyn, her friend's lodger, was carrying the casket. Alisoun found herself admiring his *so clene and faire* legs and feet. They had previously enjoyed *daliance* or flirtation while Alisoun's fourth husband was alive.[7]

The Church had much to say on the topic of sex. Intercourse that was not between a husband and wife, in the missionary position, and intended for procreation was frowned on. In addition, intercourse was forbidden even for married couples during Lent, Advent and Pentecost; on feast days; on Sundays, Wednesdays and Fridays; during menstruation, pregnancy and lactation; and for forty or so days after giving birth. The Church did not deny that a married couple had a right to sexual pleasure, albeit only because, as noted above, it was deemed necessary to conceive a child.[8] It was often held that a married couple owed each other a 'marital debt', i.e. an obligation to have sex. Thomas Mareschal confessed in 1344 that he had had an affair with his sister-in-law before he married Isabella Foxle, and had received no dispensation and therefore committed incest when he married Isabella. Pope Clement VI told Isabella that she was 'freed from the conjugal debt' as a result of her husband's actions, though it transpired that she was 'too modest to exact' the debt from him anyway. The marital debt was something each spouse owed to the other, not something deemed to apply only to men being owed sex from their wives. In 1472, Pope Sixtus IV declared that Thomas Lessy of London, who married Agnes Cokkeson and consummated the marriage but subsequently left her, had deprived Agnes of her conjugal debt.[9]

Virginity and Chastity

In the Middle Ages, 'virgin' was a word almost inevitably used of women and girls, not boys and men, and, as is the case in numerous societies, far greater emphasis was placed on the need for women to remain virgins until marriage than on men. It was taken for granted that women of high rank were virgins when they wed: when two of Edward I's daughters, Joan and Margaret, married in 1290, the Westminster chronicler called them 'noble virgins' (*virgines generosas*). And many medieval women took a vow of chastity after they were widowed, in some cases so that they could not be forced into remarriage. Although the Magna Carta stated that 'No widow shall be forced to marry so long as she wishes to live without a husband', if a widow was wealthy and therefore a desirable marriage partner, and if a king or lord was determined, he could put considerable pressure on her.[10] Mere weeks after Edward II's niece Elizabeth de Burgh was widowed from her second husband Theobald Verdon in July 1316, Edward sent her a menacing letter in which he declared that he would not be a 'good lord' to her if she did not do what he wished: marry his current favourite and perhaps lover, Roger Damory. Edward was not only Elizabeth's liege lord but her closest living male relative, and she had little choice but to bow to his demand and marry Damory. She was widowed for the third time in March 1322 at the age of twenty-six, and lived for almost four decades as a widow; she took a vow of chastity sometime before 1343 and died in November 1360.[11] Although second and third marriages were common, many landowning women preferred to live as widows and to take a vow of chastity, because they could remain in the secular world and still retain control of their own lands (when they were married, their husbands assumed control).

Widows who took this vow wore 'a certain habit', i.e. like a nun, and a ring 'in token of perpetual chastity'.[12] Eleanor, Countess of Pembroke and Leicester (1215–75), was the youngest child of King John and Isabelle of Angoulême, and Henry III's sister. Eleanor came to regret the vow of chastity she had taken before the Archbishop of Canterbury in 1231 as the teenaged widow of the Earl of Pembroke, when in early 1238 she wished to marry Simon de Montfort, a French nobleman who moved to England in c. 1230 and became Earl of Leicester. She did marry Montfort and they had six children together, as vows of chastity were reversible. Alice Hoton of the diocese of Durham lost her husband William when she was about twenty-six, and, 'pierced with grief', took a vow and wore the usual cloak and ring. In 1449, however, she petitioned the pope on the grounds that 'she might find it difficult to resist attempts to ravish her', and furthermore, that she wished to have children. Pope Nicholas V ordered the Bishop of Durham to release her from the vow and to allow her to contract a second marriage. Margaret Slengesby of

Yorkshire was allowed to commute her vow of chastity to 'other works of piety' in 1403, 'inasmuch as she fears that on account of the frailty of the flesh she will not be able to keep it, and therefore desires to marry'.[13]

Although changing one's mind was possible, the attitude towards women who did so could be negative. Pope Sixtus IV spoke in 1482 of the 'woman's levity' with which Margaret Bothe took a vow of continence after her first husband died, and afterwards changed her mind and married again, 'fearing that under the stimulus of the flesh she might give way to temptation'. And not all men respected vows, particularly when a widow was rich. Alice de Lacy was, as previously noted, forcibly married to Hugh Frene shortly after she took a vow of chastity following the death of her much-loved second husband Eble Lestrange. Benedict XII ordered the Bishop of Lincoln to subject Alice to 'spiritual penalties' for breaking her vow, as though she had done so voluntarily.[14] Sometime before July 1352, Margaret Lestrange lost her husband Hamo, and took a 'solemn vow of chastity' and entered the order of Minoresses, i.e. Franciscan nuns. She arranged with Edward III that she would enfeoff him with the lands of her inheritance, but while Sir Robert Kendale, a knight of the royal household, was escorting her to court, he 'ravished' her on Kinver Heath in Staffordshire. The king ordered the Earl of Arundel and another man to investigate.[15]

In 1447, Elizabeth Holm of York was in her sixties, and had no children with her husband of many years, Peter Percy. Furthermore, they had not cohabited or had intimate relations for about eight years. The couple, therefore, decided to 'live in chastity and devote [themselves] to holy meditations'.[16] Chaste marriage was promoted, and the example of Edward the Confessor, the king of England who died in 1066 and was canonised a century later, and who was believed to have lived chastely with his wife Edith Godwinsdaughter, was popular. Some modern writers have speculated that Richard II had a chaste marriage with his first wife Anne of Bohemia, and the fact that his second wife Isabelle de Valois was a little girl of not quite seven years old when he married her perhaps gives weight to the notion that Richard was uninterested in intercourse with women. It is certainly true that Richard and Anne had no children, but this is far more likely to have been a result of one or both partners being infertile or sub-fertile. In 1382 and again in 1383, Richard talked of his and Anne's future children, 'when God gives them', so it seems that the teenage couple had an intimate marital relationship which the king expected to result in offspring. Some years later, Queen Anne sent a letter to her brother stating that she grieved over the fact that she had not yet given birth, and in the last months of her life, aged twenty-eight, purchased herbs strongly associated with fertility and conception, such as water of plantain, trisandali, spikenard and trifera magna.[17]

Some men tried to impose chastity on their widows after their deaths by willing shops or homes to them only on condition that the women remained unmarried and chaste. If they did remarry or became intimate with another man, they would lose possession of the property. In August 1328, William Braye left his house in London to his wife Alice 'so long as she remains in pure widowhood'. Alice, however, decided to marry Nicholas Brokhurst, and in February 1345 was evicted by Juliane Braye, her late husband's niece.[18] Andrew Staunford left houses to his wife Emma and their son John in October 1319, but if Emma married again or 'knew any man carnally', John would become the houses' sole owner. In his will of October 1450, brewer Ralph Marke left his wife Juliana £40 in cash and two taverns 'so long as she remains chaste and unmarried'; otherwise, their daughter Joan Hill would have them.[19]

Chapter 7

Sexual Pleasure and Relationships (2)

Adultery and Pre-Marital Sex

Geoffroi de Charny stated that chivalrous knights should 'love a lady truly and honourably', and must 'guard the honour of your lady above all else, and keep secret the love itself and all the benefits and honourable rewards you derive from it'. In short, men were absolutely not to boast of their love affair or draw anyone's attention to it, because no good could come from this and great difficulties might arise. Charny thought that 'perfect joy' was to be found in 'being secretly in the company of one's lady' and that 'the most secret love is the most lasting and the truest'. Women, he said, should find great joy in seeing their lover publicly celebrated, admired and honoured for his great renown and glory in deeds of arms, and should 'love loyally, live joyfully and act honourably'.[1] Charny here was talking about pre-marital or extra-marital sex, not a relationship between a married couple.

Between 1401 and 1439, the authorities in London decided to clamp down on what they called 'immorality', and therefore arrested everyone whom they discovered committing adultery.[2] Adulterers were frequently caught and arrested in the middle of the night, either in their own home or their lover's, which gives an impression of busybody officials creeping around the London streets in the early hours, peering into windows. John Warham, chaplain of the church of St Michael Queenhithe, was found with his lover Margaret Wyver, a widow, at about three a.m. on 10 January 1427, and Ralph Wengrave, chaplain of the College of St Michael in Crooked Lane, was caught in bed with Agnes, wife of John Hebell from Southwark, between four and five in the morning on 31 October 1429. The punishment for adultery was to be put on the pillory, usually for an hour at a time on two consecutive days. The pillory was a wooden framework with holes in which the victim's head and hands were locked, and there were at least two pillories in medieval London: on Cornhill and Cheapside, both very busy, very public places. The tailor Richard Dodd was put in the pillory for three straight hours, an unusually long time, in December 1407 after acting as a 'bawd', i.e. a procuror, between his wife Margaret and a chaplain named William Langford. The chaplain Herman of Verona, apparently Italian though with a German-sounding given name, was 'taken in adultery with Agnes Bramptone, a married woman' on 13 July 1439, and on the same day, Joan Wakelyn, Margaret Hathewyke and Margery Bradlee were indicted before Mayor Stephen Broun for 'diverse acts provoking to public immorality'. Some men were also convicted of this offence: one was the brewer Thomas Chapell in May 1439. Hugh and Joan Carpenter, a married couple, were convicted of public immorality on the same day as Thomas Chapell and were both locked into the pillory for an hour.

The authorities did not care about unmarried people having sex, only if at least one partner was married, or if one was a member of the Church; they were not clamping down on fornication, but only on adultery. In November 1406, married woman Alice Gyboun was arrested for committing adultery with John Marchall, unmarried, and in August 1429, John Couper and Katherine Frensshe, both married to other people, were arrested and taken before the mayor and aldermen. Roger Cokke, unmarried, was 'taken in adultery' with Isabella, wife of John Blosme, on 28 January 1404. The authorities took a very dim view of anyone 'procuring' adultery, such as Richard Dodd, above. Agnes Tikell was accused in June 1406 of being a 'procuress' between Geoffrey Briggewater, who was unmarried, and Agnes Wyche.

According to the chronicler Thomas Walsingham, it was during the mayoralty of John Norhampton, in 1381/82, that the campaign against immorality first got underway in London. On 30 August 1389, the unmarried boatman John Kempe was caught with the married Isabella Smyth, and was arrested and taken before the mayor and aldermen. Adultery was usually a case for ecclesiastical courts, not for the secular authorities, but John Norhampton made it punishable by the mayor's court.[3] The chaplain William Stofford was found on 20 January 1389 to have had an affair with Alice Hoo, and they were both arrested and imprisoned. The next day, they were taken before the mayor, Nicholas Twyford, and it was proclaimed that 'if anyone wished to prosecute them, right should be done'. Nobody did, so the two sheriffs of London took William and Alice to the Consistory, the legal court of the Bishop of London, 'according to the ancient custom in dealing with priests, secular or religious, and married persons when taken in adultery in the City'.[4]

In 1400, in the area of South Wales called the Englishry, a priest named Richard Clement was hired by an unnamed male resident of the town to live in his house for a while. The man wished Richard to catch out a female relative, also unnamed, who lived in his house and whom he suspected of having illicit sexual relations. One night, she left the house 'at the repeated instigation of a married man ... for the purpose of fornication'. Richard 'followed them with sword and bow to bring her back', but was spotted by William Wellys, a servant of the married man. In the ensuing scuffle, both Clement and Wellys were wounded.[5] Also around 1400, Sir John Colvyle (b. c. 1365/69) of East Anglia had a long-term extra-marital relationship with Emma Gedeneye, and eventually arranged her marriage to a member of his household, William Talmage. John was unable or unwilling, however, to cease his relations with his lover, and often slept with Emma while she was married. When the matter came to the Bishop of Ely's attention, he realised that John Colvyle and William Talmage were related in the third and fourth degrees of kindred, but no dispensation had been issued (see the chapter 'Incest and Consanguinity' below for why this was necessary). Emma and William's marriage was annulled, and afterwards, John Colvyle and Emma decided to plight their troth and marry.[6] Either Emma had not been of high enough status for John to wish to marry or he was already married to another woman, but after he arranged her marriage to a member of his entourage he came to regret not wedding her himself, and subsequently did so. There remain unanswered questions, such as who brought the matter to the bishop's attention and why, and who knew of John Colvyle and William Talmage's familial relationship when they themselves did not know of it. The unfortunate William's feelings on the matter were unrecorded. John founded a chapel, later a college, at Saltmarsh in 1404, and statutes of the college issued in 1454 specified that Mass was to be sung for the souls of Sir John Colvyle and his wife Emma.[7]

Robert Talbott and his lover Eleanor Cantour admitted to the Bishop of Ely in 1476 that they had had frequent sexual relations for three years while Eleanor's husband was alive, and further, that Robert was the real father of several of Eleanor's children. Her husband was now dead, but they were adamant that they had not wished for his death nor done anything to bring it about. Pope Sixtus IV absolved them of adultery and stated that if they now wished to marry, he permitted it, and declared any future children legitimate. A similar case happened in 1429 between John Kupping and Margery Lomnoure of Norwich, who were lovers during the lifetime of Margery's husband and promised to marry each other once he was dead.[8]

Famous royal mistresses of the later Middle Ages include Alice Perrers, who had a long relationship with Edward III in the 1360s and 1370s – both during Edward's marriage to Philippa of Hainault and after the queen's death in 1369 – and Elizabeth 'Jane' Shore, mistress of Edward IV. Edward III and Queen Philippa's son John of Gaunt had a long relationship with Katherine Swynford during his second marriage to Constanza of Castile, and a chronicler called Gaunt a 'great fornicator' (*magnus fornicator*). Eleanor of Lancaster (d. 1372), daughter of the Earl of Lancaster and a great-granddaughter of Henry III, had a relationship with the Earl of Arundel before she married him in early 1345, almost certainly after she was widowed from Lord Beaumont in May 1342 but while Arundel was still married to her cousin Isabella Despenser.

A rather intriguing letter from Pope Innocent VI, sent to England in 1358, still exists, and states:

> A certain powerful man contracted marriage with a great and powerful lady, knowing that she was related in the third degree of kindred [i.e. second cousins] to a woman whom he had carnally known. As scandal would arise if they were separated, inasmuch as both ladies are of the magnates of the realm, and it is expedient that the matter should be secret and not published by letters or otherwise, the pope is prayed to commit the matter verbally to the cardinal of Albano for dispensation.[9]

It is unfortunate that the people in question, all of them from the highest levels of society, were not identified. Henry, Duke of Lancaster, wrote in 1354 that common women were more responsive to his touch than noblewomen, and the fact that he had points of comparison suggests that he had pre-marital or extra-marital experience with noblewomen, and not only with his wife Isabella Beaumont. In 1312, the Archbishop

Sexual Pleasure and Relationships (2)

of York, William Greenfield, charged Sir Gerard Salvayn and Margaret, wife of Sir Robert Percy, with adultery, and in the same year declared that Paulina, the wife of Sir John Graas, was committing adultery with Sir Richard Waleys and living in his house.[10] The July 1254 inquisition post mortem of Isabel 'Sibyl' Brok, called 'the lady of Chetinton' (Chetton in Shropshire), stated that she had had sisters Alice, Edelina and Clemence, now dead, and that Clemence had already been pregnant with her eldest son Auger when she married William Maleseveres. Her three younger sons, Thomas, Simon and Adam, were 'begotten in matrimony'. Auger's last name was Tatlinton, not Maleseveres, but although he was evidently the son of his mother's lover and not her husband, in February 1256 he was found to be one of the three heirs of his aunt Sibyl, and made an excellent marriage to Emma Luttleton, lady of Frankley.[11]

Margaret Gatesden of Sussex was born in the mid-thirteenth century as the daughter and heir of Sir John Gatesden and Hawise Nevill. She married Sir John Camoys (c. 1250–98) and had a son, Ralph, Lord Camoys, in the early 1270s (Ralph was at least twenty-one in 1294, and died in 1335). In or before 1277, Margaret fell in love with another man, Sir William Paynel, left her husband, and went to live with William. John Camoys' reaction was one of astonishing benevolence and kindness: he issued a deed on 11 June 1285 stating that 'I will and grant ... that the aforesaid Margaret is to live and remain with the aforesaid Sir William', transferred his rights to the greater part of Margaret's inheritance to Paynel, and gave up his claims to her goods and chattels. In 1300, it was stated that Margaret 'lived with the same William ... with the consent and by the will of the said John, then the husband of the same Margaret'. John Camoys died shortly before 4 June 1298, and Margaret married William Paynel in or before 1300. Edward I's government claimed after John died that she had no right to dower as John's widow because she had 'abandoned' him, was 'guilty of the crime of adultery', and 'is living in adultery rather than in any other proper or lawful manner'.

Gilbert St Leofard, Bishop of Chichester, however, acknowledged that in early 1296 Margaret had 'solemnly and canonically purged herself' of adultery before Gilbert's dean and treasurer, the prioress of Easebourne, four named ladies, and 'many other married woman and young maidens [*domicellas*] of the neighbourhood'. The bishop, therefore, declared her innocent of the crime and requested that she might be restored to her good name. William Paynel had also 'legally purged himself' of adultery before John Pecham, Archbishop of Canterbury, in 1288.[12] The reaction of Edward I's government to the Margaret Gatesden situation mentions 'a recent statute concerning women leaving their husbands and living with their adulterers and not reconciled freely and without ecclesiastical coercion before the deaths of their husbands ... in which it is expressly contained that, if a wife freely leaves her husband and goes to live with her adulterer, she is to lose in perpetuity her action for claiming her dower which might belong to her' (this was the Second Statute of Westminster in 1285; see also Chapter 3 above).

Emma Snave was a few months pregnant when she married Stephen Herryngg in Kent in early 1285 – their wedding took place just after the Epiphany, i.e. 6 January – and gave birth to her son John on 22 March. Whether John was Stephen's son is not clear.[13] Roger Longe, a vintner of London, made his will on 29 September 1375 and died before 14 January 1376. He left money to Maud Beccote or Bectote, presumably a relative, friend, neighbour or servant, 'if she be *enceinte* in the opinion of his executors'. Maud was indeed pregnant, and died soon after giving birth: on 2 August 1376, her daughter Isabel, aged six months, was given into the custody of Adam Meryfeld, a goldsmith. Adam was presumably Maud's lover and Isabel's father, though this was not specifically stated. Maud Beccote was not married when Roger Longe made his will, as he left her £20 as her future dowry and gave her a further twenty marks (3,200d) for her 'uterine child'. After Maud's death, this money was also given into the custody of Adam Meryfeld to look after until little Isabel came of age. Maud became pregnant outside marriage, though there is no hint of judgement on Roger Longe's part, perhaps because Roger himself had an illegitimate son called John, as well as two sons, Thomas and William, born in wedlock.[14]

Thomas Hodyng of Liston in Essex, aged thirty-three, had an affair with Agnes, his father's 'maidservant', which resulted in the birth of a son also named Thomas in June 1336. What subsequently happened to Agnes was not explained, though her son Thomas was still alive twenty-one years later.[15] Joan Gade of London had an illegitimate son with William Beneyt, and in 1365 accused him of killing the boy and of threatening her, even though he had promised to marry her. William produced the boy alive in court.[16] Maud Flete had a relationship with William Spark of London, who died in July 1379, which resulted in an illegitimate son named Robert sometime before April 1361.[17] Before she married her husband Walter Lillebrok in or before 1353, Eleanor Wynston had a sexual relationship with a man, name not recorded, who was Walter's kinsman, and in 1406, Richard Welle and Christina Bockan of the diocese of Durham married after they committed 'fornication' and long after they had several children together.[18]

Unchaste Ecclesiastics

Walter Langton, Bishop of Coventry and Lichfield and treasurer of England (d. 1321), was accused at the beginning of the 1300s of having committed adultery with Joan Briançon while her husband Sir John Lovetot (d. 1294) was alive. After Lovetot's death, the bishop supposedly kept Joan as his concubine, and she accompanied him everywhere. Lovetot's son John Lovetot the younger, Joan's stepson, even accused her of strangling his father while in bed with him, at the behest of her lover the bishop. 'All these matters are publicly known in England and by the English at [the papal court in] Rome,' Lovetot announced, though Pope Boniface VIII and Robert Winchelsey, Archbishop of Canterbury, found Langton innocent.[19] The word 'concubine', *concubina* in Latin, was used in the Middle Ages to refer to women who, like Joan Briançon, were believed to have had sexual relations with a churchman.[20] Pope Martin V thundered in 1423 about William Beache, abbot of Buckfast in Devon, who 'has begotten children by diverse women whom he keeps as concubines'.[21]

In 1405, Pope Innocent VII ordered the archdeacon of Taunton and a canon of Wells to go to the Benedictine monastery of Wintney, Hampshire. Its prioress for the last twenty years, Alice, 'cherishes two immodest nuns', one of whom was her sister, who had apostatised and left the monastery and had given birth to children. The other nun remained at the monastery, but lived 'in evil life and lewdness'. Prioress Alice herself had taken a secular priest called Thomas Ferring as her 'companion at board and in bed' (wording which implies marriage). Ferring had his own chamber within the monastery, contrary to regulations, and Alice went there day and night 'to satisfy their lust'. The archdeacon and canon were to remove her from the monastery if they found the story to be true, owing to the 'enormous and scandalous crimes' Alice had committed. A few decades later, Elizabeth Broke, abbess of Romsey Abbey in Hampshire, admitted that she had 'recently allowed herself to be carnally known, whereby she fears that she is pregnant', and in 1424 it transpired that Cecily Marmyll, a nun of Amesbury Priory in Wiltshire, had given birth to two children from relationships with two secular priests.[22] Margaret Grenefeld, nun of Amesbury Priory in Wiltshire, 'allowed herself to be seduced by an unmarried man' and bore a child after she entered the priory in 1397, and in 1403 John Holmborn, monk of Robertsbridge in Sussex, was beaten on the orders of his abbot after being found having sex with a woman in a wood.[23] In October 1328, John Cales, a chaplain of Jersey in the Channel Islands, petitioned Edward III about the rightful inheritance of the eight illegitimate children he had fathered with a woman named Reginalda; their names were John, Peter, Philip, William, Philipota, Guilimota, Raolina and Simonetta.[24]

In 2019, archivists unearthed the fascinating story of a nun named Joan of Leeds in a record book of William Melton (d. 1340), Archbishop of York. Bored of life in the convent of St Clement's in York, Joan faked a serious illness and her own death, and persuaded several of her fellow nuns to inter a lifesize dummy of her in consecrated ground. Now officially dead and buried, Joan moved to Beverley thirty miles away. Archbishop Melton, after the fake burial was discovered in 1318, sent a letter to the dean of Beverley saying that Joan had 'perverted her path of life arrogantly to the way of carnal lust ... she now wanders at large to the notorious peril of her soul'. Nor was this St Clement's first scandal: in 1300/01, a nun, Cecily, left the convent with a group of men late one evening and rode with them to Darlington. Here she lived with her lover, Gregory Thornton, for more than three years. This escape had, like Joan's, obviously been well planned.[25]

Unchaste priests in London, if caught with a woman, were to be imprisoned in a jail called the Tun, and a third offence would result in banishment from London. His partner would be arraigned in the Guildhall before the mayor and sheriffs, sent to Newgate prison where her head would be shaved, and taken from there to the Tun accompanied by minstrels (i.e. to make a song and dance to draw public attention to her).[26] The 1386 case of Elizabeth Moring, a brothel-keeper banished from London, revealed that she forced her female servants 'to consort with friars, chaplains, and all other such men as desired to have their company' (see also Chapter 13 below).[27] There is much evidence that chaplains, though members of the Church, often behaved astonishingly badly, and it is remarkable how many were caught in the London

Sexual Pleasure and Relationships (2)

authorities' clampdown on immorality in the early 1400s. In June 1300, Ralph, a chaplain who lived in Portsoken ward in London, 'was a receiver of thieves and prostitutes', chaplain Richard Despenser was in a relationship in 1305 with Juliane Hoddere, called his 'concubine', and in February 1326 chaplain Alan Hacford stabbed Walter Anne in the stomach and killed him after finding Walter in bed with Alice of York, who was also Alan's lover. In November 1387, Margaret Morys of Loddon in Norfolk discovered that she was pregnant by the local chaplain, Thomas Holm, and 'for shame took her goods on the following day and left the town'. Exactly a century earlier on Christmas Day 1287, Hugh Weston, chaplain of Acton Scott, Shropshire, was drunk after sunset, and got into a quarrel with some men singing outside a tavern. One of them was John Querebus, whom Hugh hated 'because he sang well, and because he [Hugh] desired the love of certain women standing by in a field'. To impress the women, Hugh attacked John with a sword, and almost cut two fingers off his left hand.[28] Misbehaving and unchaste chaplains and priests were not punished with the pillory like other people, but were sent to the local bishop's court. Numerous popes granted dispensations to 'persons of illegitimate birth, even the sons of priests' to be ordained into the Church, so evidently, it was not uncommon for priests to father children.[29] A man who died in Northamptonshire in 1323 was called John le Personesone, which means 'the parson's son', and he himself 'kept one Amice as a concubine' and had two illegitimate sons with her.[30]

Chapter 8

Love Language

Although we have no diaries and only very few personal letters from the Middle Ages, we do have poems. Middle English literature often dealt with courtly love, and the songs of the French troubadours provided inspiration for English poets; the woman who is the object of the poet's unrequited love is beautiful and virtuous, and forever out of reach.[1] The Middle English word *leman* or *lemmon*, meaning one's lover or sweetheart, was a unisex word, and appears in a poem written in the late thirteenth or early fourteenth century which now bears the title *Fairest Between Lincoln and Lindsey*:

> *Ich have loved all this yer* [year]
> *That I may love na more;*
> *Ich have siked mony sik* [sighed many sighs],
> *Lemmon, for thine ore* [your favour].
> *Me nis love never the ner* [love is not nearer to me],
> *And that me reweth sore* [grieves me greatly].
> *Swete lemmon, thench on me* [think about me]:
> *Ich have loved thee yore* [a long time].
>
> *Swete lemmon, I preye thee* [pray you]
> *Of love one speche* [for one word of love].
> *Whil I live, in world so wide*
> *Other nulle I seche* [I will not seek another].
> *With thy love, my swete lef* [dear],
> *My blis thou mightes eche* [you might increase my bliss]:
> *A swete kos* [kiss] *of thy mouth*
> *Mighte be my leche* [leech, i.e. letting blood might cure me].[2]

A poem now called *A Cleric Courts His Lady*, also from the late thirteenth or early fourteenth century, says *Whet helpeth thee, my swete lemman/My lif thus for to gaste?* (What do you gain, my sweet lover, to make my life anguished like this?)[3] The song *Byrd one Brere* or 'Bird on a briar' dates from c. 1290 to 1320, though the words and music were written on the back of a papal bull dating to 1199. It contains the lyrics:

> *Hic am so blithe, so bryhit, brid on brere,*
> *Quan I se that hende in halle:*
> *Yhe is whit of lime, loveli, trewe*
> *Yhe is fayr and flur of alle.*
> *Mikte ic hire at wille haven,*
> *Stedefast of love, loveli, trewe,*
> *Of mi sorwe yhe may me saven*
> [I am so blithe, so bright, bird on a briar,
> When I see that handmaid in the hall:
> She is white of limb, lovely, true;
> She is fair, and the flower of all.
> Might I have her at my will,
> Steadfast of love, lovely, true,
> Of my sorrow she may save me][4]

Geoffrey Chaucer's *Parlement of Fowles*, 'Parliament of Fowls' in modern spelling and literally meaning 'the talking of birds', shows that Valentine's Day was already celebrated in the late fourteenth century. In the poem, a group of birds meet to choose their mates for the coming year on *seynt valentynes day*. One of the Paston Letters, dated 1477, is the earliest extant example of a lover being called a 'Valentine': Margery Brews addressed her fiancé John Paston as 'my right well beloved Valentine John Paston' and 'right reverent and worshipful and my right well beloved Valentine'.[5]

In modern English, the words 'have sex', 'make love' and even 'fuck' can be used by both men and women and are actions someone does *with* someone else; they do not have to indicate that someone, inevitably a man, does something *to* someone. A woman can say 'I want to fuck you' to a man or another woman just as easily as a man can say it to a woman. Ruth Mazo Karras points out that the same is not true in medieval usage, and indeed, the Middle English Dictionary translates the medieval equivalent of 'fuck', *swive(n)*, as either 'to have sexual intercourse' or 'to have sexual intercourse with a woman'. In modern French, *foutre* means 'to fuck' and can, like the English word, be used by and about both men and women, but in medieval French, as Karras says, it meant 'to penetrate' and the person who penetrated could only be a man. There are other, similar medieval words relating to intercourse where the man is the subject, the active partner who does, and the woman is the object, the passive partner who is done to.[6] And to give another example, a papal dispensation was granted in 1353 which allowed Walter Lillebrok and Eleanor Wynston to remain married, even though Walter was related to a man who had 'carnally known Eleanor'.[7] The unnamed man here is positioned as the active agent who 'knew' a woman, while Eleanor is the passive subject who was 'known' by a man.

It is rare to find a reference in a household account to lovemaking, though one of Edward II's accounts in October 1324 states that the king crossed the River Thames from the Tower of London to a house he had rented in Southwark called La Rosere. In another example of the gendered language which Ruth Mazo Karras discusses, the king's extant account now held in the National Archives states that Edward *fist p[ri]uement son deduyt a cele place*, 'secretly took his pleasure in that place' or 'privately made love in that place'.[8] *Faire son deduit* (or *deduyt* or *dedoit*) is translated in the online Anglo-Norman Dictionary as 'to have one's pleasure (of a woman)'.[9] Given the debate about Edward II's sexuality over the last 700 years, and the frequent modern assumption that he was gay and uninterested in women, it is rather intriguing to note that the secret lover with whom the forty-year-old king made love in 1324 was evidently a woman.

Euphemisms were sometimes used in medieval literature: Geoffrey Chaucer's Wife of Bath refers to her private parts as *my bele chose*, 'my fair thing', and elsewhere states that she *hadde the beste quoniam* [that] *myghte be* and calls it her *chambre of Venus*. In his *Book of Holy Medicines*, Henry of Grosmont, Duke of Lancaster, used the word 'kiss', *beiser* in the Anglo-Norman original, as a euphemism to describe what he did with women. In modern French, *un baiser* means 'a kiss' while *baiser* as a verb means 'to fuck'. 'Incontinent' was often used as a euphemism for a person who could not or would not control their lust, and in the medieval French often used in English documents, prostitutes were called *femmes de fole vie* or 'women of lewd life', another common euphemism. Chaucer's bawdy and farcical *Miller's Tale*, by contrast, uses deliberately earthy language. Nicholas, the clerk who lusts after his landlord's young wife Alisoun, makes his feelings known to her in a very physical way: *he caughte hire by the queynte*, i.e. her private parts, and exclaims '*Lemman, love me al atones or I wol dyen*', 'Sweetheart, love me immediately or I will die'.

Peter Taverner of London was called a *holer*, meaning adulterer or fornicator, in 1311, and in 1321 William Counte also of London was nicknamed *Frelove* or 'free love'.[10] It is surely not a coincidence that William's second name means either 'count' or 'cunt', which in Middle English was spelt *cunte, conte, counte*, or, as in the *Miller's Tale* quoted above, *queynte* or *queinte*. The name of Gropecuntelane, one of the places in London where the sex trade took place, meant exactly the same thing 700 years ago that it means today, and another medieval word was *cunte-beten* (beaten), meaning impotent.[11] Other modern English words relating to sex and body parts have a long history as well, such as 'bollocks', which is recorded as *balloks* in the fourteenth century. The origin of the word 'fuck' is surprisingly obscure; it is first certainly recorded with its modern meaning around 1475, and most probably entered English from Low German, Dutch or Frisian.[12] The idea one sometimes sees shared online, that the word is an acronym for Fornication Under Consent of the King or For Unlawful Carnal Knowledge, is nonsense. Adam Fuckere and his sons Adam, William and John were accused of assault in Somerset in 1315, and one of Edward I's palfreymen of 1286 bore the last name Fuckebeggere. In the thirteenth and fourteenth centuries, the word probably meant 'to strike' rather than its modern meaning.[13]

One exception to the general lack of medieval writing on sexual matters is the late fifteenth-century verse 'A Talk of Ten Wives on their Husbands' Ware'. The women sit in a tavern, and because they have nothing else to talk about, discuss their husbands' privates. The second wife stated that she met her husband '*[w]hen he was in his moste pryde*', i.e. in his greatest glory, '*[t]he lenghte of thre bene*' (length of three beans). Another woman's husband's penis was the '*lenghte of a snayle*' (snail), and another complained that her husband '*pysses his tarse every yere*', i.e. only ejaculated once a year. The sixth wife's spouse was impotent and his penis *lythe styll* despite her efforts to arouse him, and the seventh's was a '*sory pyne* [sorry pin] *that schuld hengge bytwen his leggis*' but instead was '*a sory laveroke satt on brode opon two adyll eggis*', a sorry lark sitting on a nest on two addled eggs.[14]

Chapter 9

Pregnancy and Childbirth (1)

Menstruation

It seems probable that the average onset of menstruation, the menarche, occurred at a rather later age than is the case in modern industrialised societies. The *Trotula* stated that menses should begin 'around the thirteenth year, or a little earlier or a little later, depending on the degree to which they [girls] have an excess or dearth of heat or cold'.[1] Medieval England followed Pliny's belief that menstrual blood was dangerous not only to menstruating women themselves but to everything else; contact with menstrual blood turned new wine sour, crops would become barren, and dogs who tasted it died of rabies. Intercourse during menstruation was to be avoided at all costs, as any child thus conceived would have red hair and would contract leprosy.[2]

The authors of the *Trotula* believed that women menstruate because there was 'not enough heat in women to dry up the bad and superfluous humours' in them, and because their physical weakness compared to men meant that women were unable to tolerate physical exercise sufficient to expel these humours. The *Trotula* detailed treatments for menstrual issues. For delayed menstruation, the roots of the red willow were recommended: they were to be pulverised, mixed with wine or water and cooked, and drunk in the morning when the mixture was lukewarm. Another solution was to bleed the woman from a vein on the sole of her foot. Heavy periods were, rather hilariously, to be cured with a mixture of pennyroyal, laurel leaves and the 'soles of old shoes' cooked together. Alternatively, hot ashes could be mixed with hot red wine and made into a dough, wrapped into a piece of linen cloth, and inserted into the vagina.[3]

Conception and Contraception

Except for women and girls who wished to live a religious life and who were veiled at a religious house, the general expectation was that women would marry and have children. Ruth Mazo Karras has pointed out that '[m]otherhood was the one role for women that most medieval people held as a norm'.[4] The *Trotula* recognised that some women had difficulty conceiving a child, and put this down to them being too thin, or too fat, or having a womb 'too slippery and smooth'. Sometimes men were deemed at fault by the *Trotula*'s writers for having 'excessively thin seed' or 'extremely dry and cold testicles', and the notion that men might be infertile and that a couple's childlessness was not necessarily the woman's fault was an unusual one in the Middle Ages. Its suggestion to couples to discover which of them was infertile was to fill two pots with wheat bran and to put the man's urine in one pot and the woman's in the other. The pot containing the urine of the infertile partner would stink and be full of worms after a few days. If a woman wished to conceive a boy, her husband needed to find a female hare, extract its womb and vagina, make a powder of them, and put the powder in wine and drink it. The woman herself needed to do the same thing with the testicles of a male hare, and was then to have intercourse with her husband at the end of her next period. Alternatively, to conceive a boy, a woman should lie with her left hip higher than her right after intercourse, so that her husband's seed would naturally fall to the right, where males were conceived. If she wished for a daughter, she should lie with her right hip higher than the left. To conceive a child of either sex, it was recommended to take the testicles of an uncastrated male pig or wild boar, dry them, and for the woman to swallow the powder with some wine.[5]

Although it was taken for granted that most women would become mothers or least wished to, there were of course occasions when women did not want to become pregnant. Because of the medieval idea that the fetus was not considered to be alive until it quickened or 'ensouled', the difference between contraception and abortion was not as clear-cut as it is today.[6] For women who wished not to conceive, the *Trotula* recommended placing the womb of a goat that had never had offspring against her naked flesh, presumably while having intercourse. Alternatively, she could remove a weasel's testicles and carry them on her bosom, wrapped in goose skin.[7] This seems only likely to work as a contraceptive because her partner would find trying to make love with a woman in the presence of dead animal flesh deeply off-putting, and the most effective medieval methods of preventing conception were coitus interruptus or abstinence. Herbs used to induce miscarriages, meanwhile, were rue and sage drunk with water.[8]

Miscarriages and Abortions

Sometime before December 1304 on Guernsey in the Channel Islands, Matilda Bonamy, also known as Matilda du Val, became pregnant from a pre-marital relationship with Jordan Dorree, also known as Jordan Cloyet or Clouet. Matilda suggested that they marry, which, if the ceremony took place before the birth, would ensure the legitimacy of the child. Jordan refused, so Matilda took the matter to the local bishop's court, and Jordan was excommunicated. Matilda was given letters pertaining to her lover's excommunication, and when a furious Jordan encountered her carrying them, he reacted violently, and shoved her to the ground. Matilda went into premature labour and her child was stillborn, and she herself died shortly afterwards. Accused of the murder of his former lover and their unborn child, Jordan sought sanctuary in a church in St Peter Port and then fled from the Channel Islands, though Edward I pardoned him in December 1304 on the grounds that he slew the child in Matilda's womb by accident and not by malice aforethought. The matter was still under discussion seventeen years later in January 1322, when Edward II stated, rather puzzlingly, that Jordan merely consented to the murder of Matilda and her unborn child, and in fact, it was his sister Emma who killed them. On this occasion, the child 'whom the said Matilda brought forth abortively' was said to be a boy, while Jordan himself was still alive in 1322 and apparently thriving.[9]

Deliberately bringing about miscarriage or premature labour by assaulting a woman was, in medieval England and elsewhere in Europe, a felony punishable by death. The fetus was deemed to have acquired a soul at the time of 'quickening' around the fourth month (i.e. when a woman first feels the fetus stirring), and killing it after this stage, though not before, was deemed homicide. In the mid-thirteenth century, Henry Bracton composed a work in Latin called *On the Laws and Customs of England*, and stated 'If one strikes a pregnant woman or gives her poison in order to procure an abortion, if the fetus is already formed or quickened, especially if it is quickened, he commits homicide.' An anonymous treatise called *Fleta*, dating from around 1290, confirms that a person was guilty of homicide if he struck a woman or gave her poison, thereby 'not allowing conception' or causing an abortion (*faciat abortivum*). This also applied to a pregnant woman who deliberately drank something to destroy the 'quickened child' she carried. In his book *Eve's Herbs*, John Riddle cites the case of Richard Bourton of Bristol, who in the 1320s beat a woman named Alice while she was heavily pregnant with twins. Soon afterwards, Alice gave birth to one dead infant and one who was born alive but died two days later. Bourton was tried before the King's Bench, though was pardoned by Edward III in May 1327.[10]

William Ammory broke into the London home of a 'poor woman', Emma Whitewell, who was pregnant, on Ash Wednesday in 1355. He assaulted her 'so violently and in so horrible a manner' that she gave birth prematurely to a stillborn infant and was bedridden for seven weeks. A jury, however, acquitted Ammory of wrongdoing.[11] On 29 September 1326, Sir Piers Denarston and a group of his men attacked the home of his neighbours John and Emma Neve in Brent Eleigh, Suffolk, and stole livestock and goods. The furious John Neve claimed that Denarston's men defiled Emma, who was heavily pregnant, and frightened her so much that 'the child within her stomach perished'. A similar attack took place in May 1406. Lord Zouche (b. c. 1373) attacked the Bedfordshire home of his stepmother Lady Arundel, with whom he was feuding, and caused her pregnant daughter-in-law Elizabeth Talbot, wife of Zouche's stepbrother John Arundel (b. 1385), to go into premature labour. The infant died, and Lady Arundel's petition to Henry IV stated that Elizabeth 'lay in peril of death' as well; as the young woman is known to have died in 1406, it seems that the ordeal did indeed kill her. Lord Zouche, a peer of the realm, was summoned to parliament to explain himself, though he was not executed and lived until 1415.[12]

One night at the end of March 1301, John Sherman and Augustine Curzon broke into the London home of Adam and Alice Cobel. They launched a brutal attack on Adam after he discovered them ransacking his home, and when Alice tried to protect her husband, they assaulted her too. Alice was pregnant, and gave birth to a premature child soon after the attack. She never recovered from her injuries, and died two months later on 31 May; Sherman and Curzon fled, and the sheriffs ordered their arrest. Another pregnant woman attacked in London was Lucy, wife of Richard Barstaple, beaten and kicked to the ground by Agnes Houdydoudy in late June 1326. Lucy gave birth prematurely to a dead infant three weeks later and herself died a month after the attack. Agnes was caught and imprisoned in Newgate, and perhaps was later executed, though records are missing. And finally, shortly before

1340, clerk Richard Wegenholt of Pulham Market in Norfolk kicked Alice Couper while she was pregnant. Alice gave birth to a premature daughter, Joan, who died immediately after baptism with 'the injury of the blow being manifest in her side'. Wegenholt was arrested and imprisoned in Norwich, accused of homicide, but 'purged his innocence' before Anthony Bek, Bishop of Norwich (d. 1343).[13] Whatever the law said, there appears to have been an extraordinary reluctance to convict and punish anyone who assaulted or attacked pregnant women.

Pennyroyal was used after miscarriages to clear the womb of any infection (though in modern times is considered too dangerous to use for this purpose) and to increase uterine contractions. An apothecary's account for Edward II's queen Isabella of France is still extant, and shows that in or soon before November 1313, pennyroyal was purchased for her. Half a pound of it cost 6d.[14] This purchase surely, therefore, reveals that Queen Isabella had suffered a miscarriage, a year after she bore her first child, Edward III, in November 1312. Edward II's mother Leonor of Castile might also have miscarried a child on 29 May 1255, less than seven months after her wedding and when she was still only thirteen years old. Many years later, Leonor marked the obituary of a daughter of hers who died in Bordeaux on 29 May, and it is difficult to determine another year when she was in Bordeaux on that date, except in 1255.[15]

The *Trotula* states that when a woman was at the start of her pregnancy, 'nothing should be named in front of her which she is not able to have, because if she sets her mind on it and is not able to have it, this occasions miscarriage'. Pica, the condition where a pregnant woman desires to eat things normally considered inedible, was known in the Middle Ages: the *Trotula* recommended that if a woman wished to eat clay, chalk or coal, she should be given beans cooked with sugar.[16]

Chapter 10

Pregnancy and Childbirth (2)

Examining Women's Bodies

Gilbert de Clare, Earl of Gloucester, eldest grandchild of Edward I, was killed at the Battle of Bannockburn in June 1314, aged twenty-three. His widow Maud – whom his envoys had chosen as the 'fairest' of the Earl of Ulster's four unmarried daughters in 1308 – claimed to be pregnant after his death, though in fact was not (or perhaps she miscarried or the infant was stillborn). Because Gilbert's vast annual income of £7,000 would pour into the coffers of his uncle Edward II for many years until his heir came of age, the king had a strong vested interest in pretending that his niece-in-law Maud would bear the late earl's child, and, astonishingly, continued this pretence for nearly three years until May 1317. Gilbert's sister Eleanor and her husband Hugh Despenser, who, with Eleanor's two younger sisters, were Gilbert's co-heirs, asked for their inheritance to be given to them in February 1316. Despenser pointed out, correctly, that 'so much time has passed that if the said countess were pregnant, according to the common course of childbirth she could not be said to have been made pregnant by the aforementioned earl'. Edward II's lawyers, however, claimed that the countess was certainly pregnant by her husband – twenty months after his death – and 'felt a living boy in her belly'. They told the couple that they should 'have the belly of the aforesaid countess inspected by knights and discreet matrons [*ad inspiciendum ventrem predicte comitisse per milites et matronas discretas*], to see whether the said countess were pregnant or not; and if so, then when she was expected to give birth'.[1]

A similar case occurred a century later, when Drew or Drogo Barentyn, formerly mayor of London, died in December 1415. His heir was his late brother Thomas's son Reynold, in his thirties, but his widow Christina claimed to be pregnant. Nicholas Wotton, the current mayor, with two other 'discreet' men and four women, were appointed to examine Christina's 'breasts and belly' (*ubera et ventrem*) to ascertain if she was truly pregnant, and if so, when the infant was expected. The seven – Mayor Wotton, Robert Chichele, William Crowmere, Elizabeth Curyell, Elizabeth Fraunceys, Rose Louth and Katherine Frenssh – established that she was not carrying Drew's posthumous child.[2] It would appear that in both 1316 and 1415, men were permitted to see and touch the bodies and private parts of the dowager Countess of Gloucester and the mayor of London's widow. In 1296, a male jury and 'certain women' examined John Wodeureton's widow Margaret to see if she was pregnant, and on 3 July 1304, six women examined another Margaret, widow of twenty-one-year-old Richard Rokele of Norfolk (d. 26 January 1304), in the presence of twelve knights; they 'say positively that she is not pregnant'.[3]

The author of an early fourteenth-century chronicle, commenting on the claimed pregnancy of the dowager Countess of Gloucester in 1314/16, stated that she 'has been expected to give birth for a year or more; and if she should now give birth, I do not see by what right the boy could claim the inheritance, because the law warns us that if a posthumous child is born after the eleventh month, it cannot claim the inheritance of the deceased'.[4] It would appear that contemporaries believed that a pregnancy might last eleven months.

Birth Aids and Customs

There were prayers and rituals designed to help women through the stress of childbearing. In his book of medicines, the *Liber receptorum medicinalium*, the English surgeon John Arderne (c. 1307–80) included a charm to help speed labour, which was to be tied below the knee of the labouring woman while saying the Lord's Prayer and the Ave Maria. The charm was a written incantation that, with Mary's intercession and Jesus's bidding, 'may you successfully give birth to the child you bear in your womb'.[5] Certain objects, notably belts or girdles once in the possession of a saint, were also believed to help women through labour. The belt and hat of Thomas, Earl of Lancaster, executed in 1322 and widely regarded in Yorkshire as an unofficial saint until the Reformation, were supposed to help women in childbirth. Two monks of Westminster Abbey took one of their most sacred relics, the girdle of the Virgin Mary, to Knaresborough in Yorkshire when Edward I's daughter Elizabeth, Countess of Hereford, gave birth to her second child there in September 1304. Henry VII's queen Elizabeth of York asked for 'our Lady gyrdelle' to be delivered to her in December 1502, a few weeks before she gave birth; perhaps this was the same girdle as the one used by the Countess of Hereford two centuries earlier.[6]

If a woman struggled in labour, the *Trotula* recommended that she take a bath in water containing mallow, fenugreek, linseed and barley, and afterwards, 'let there be a fumigation of spikenard and other aromatic substances'. Trying to make her sneeze with powder of frankincense was another option. For opening and strengthening the birth canal, white hellebore ground into a powder was recommended; alarmingly, this was believed to 'shake the organs' and help push the fetus out. After childbirth, says the *Trotula*, '[t]he womb, as though it were a wild beast of the forest, because of the sudden evacuation, falls this way and that, as if it were wandering'. As the wandering womb caused terrible pain, the *Trotula* recommended the tops of the elder plant mixed with barley flour and the white of an egg made into little wafers with suet, and warm wine with cumin. The womb could wander from its rightful place on other occasions as well, said the *Trotula*, following widespread contemporary medical opinion, and one symptom was pain in the left side.[7]

Seclusion or lying-in, the custom where a noble or royal woman spent the last few weeks of her pregnancy in a darkened room with only female attendants, appears to be a fifteenth-century development. On 2 December 1325, Edward II visited and dined with his heavily pregnant niece Eleanor Despenser at the royal manor-house of Sheen on the Thames (later Richmond Palace). She gave birth there on or before 14 December, when the king offered 30s to the Virgin Mary in gratitude that 'God granted [Eleanor] a prompt delivery of her child'.[8] Lady Despenser was obviously not in seclusion, and was able to see male relatives during the last few days of her pregnancy. There is evidence that men were even allowed in a woman's birthing chamber in the thirteenth and fourteenth centuries. William, Lord Ferrers was born at his father William the elder's manor of Groby in Leicestershire at the end of January 1272. His mother Anne's chamberlain was named Richard Frounceys, and it appears that Richard was inside the chamber when Anne gave birth: Richard stated a few years later that 'when she was in labour, Sir William Ferrers her husband came to the door of the said lady's chamber, and the said Richard opened it that his lord might come in to speak with her'. Possibly Richard was in an outer chamber, though this is not stated, and Anne's husband was allowed to come in and talk to her while she was in labour. Robert Haryngton was born in Gleaston, Lancashire (now Cumbria) on 28 March 1356, and when he proved in 1377 that he was now twenty-one and of age, servant John Grys stated that he 'was on that day in the chamber where the child was born'.[9]

Henry, Lord Percy (1273–1314) was in Leconfield, Yorkshire when his wife Eleanor Fitzalan gave birth to their son Henry there on 6 February 1301, and immediately rode twelve miles to his manor of Nafferton to inform his tenants of the good news. Katherine Whissh bore her son Henry in an upstairs chamber of her home on Brudenestret (now Staple Gardens) in Winchester, Hampshire on 24 March 1334 while her husband Henry the elder and her brother Geoffrey were downstairs in the hall. On other occasions, fathers were a few miles away when their wives gave birth. Richard Danseye's third son Walter was born in Dilton Marsh, Wiltshire in early December 1340 while Richard himself was ten miles away in Holt, fox-hunting. Richard gave 40d to William Workman who came to him and said 'My lord, do you wish to hear news?' and told him of Walter's birth the day before. Fulk Grey was on pilgrimage in Canterbury when his son Fulk the younger was born in Cambridge on 28 October 1382.[10] Bringing a father news of his son's birth could be lucrative, especially when the father was king of England: Edward II granted John Launge the huge sum of £80 annually for life for the simple act of walking from one part of Windsor Castle to another on 13 November 1312 to inform Edward that Queen Isabella had borne their son, later Edward III.[11]

Women in medieval England, or at least women who were not royal or noble, were not secluded after giving birth either, and were able to receive visitors, including men. John Leddred visited Isabel Chasteleyn two days after she bore her daughter Joan in Dinnington, Somerset in March 1348, while Isabel was still 'in her childbed'; a few months later, four other Somerset men visited Joan Denboud, also in bed, on the day she gave birth to her son John; and in Dorset in June 1335, John Watton, Robert FitzPayn and other men visited Alice Cary 'lying in childbirth' on the day she bore her son Thomas. Lettice Seynclere gave birth to her son John in Somerset in October 1355, and on the fourth day after the birth, four men visited her to 'comfort' her, and gave her son and his

Pregnancy and Childbirth (2)

nurse gifts. After Beatrice Frechevyle gave birth to Margaret, the elder of her two daughters, in Nettleworth, Nottinghamshire on 12 May 1383, villager John Ufton visited her and gave her two pheasants. Katherine Torell bore her son John in Herongate, Essex on 15 October 1423, and five local residents, Thomas Rede, John Elyot, Thomas Hulk, John Wythyr and Stephen Penyfader, 'to comfort her in her convalescence' and to express their pleasure that she had survived childbirth, visited her and brought her gifts: twelve partridges, six pheasants, eight capons, four 'fat geese' and a 'barren doe'. This occurred on the same day that Katherine gave birth.[12] Clearly there was no societal prohibition in late medieval England on men unrelated to the mother entering the bedchamber where she had borne her child and where she was recovering. On the other hand, Marguerite of Anjou, queen of Henry VI, remained in seclusion with female attendants both before and after giving birth to Edward of Lancaster in October 1453. A curtain was drawn across the queen's chamber and no men were allowed to see her until she was purified a few weeks after the birth.[13]

It was common for jurors to remember an infant's date of birth many years later, when the child had grown up and wished to claim an inheritance, because they heard the infant's mother crying out during labour. Adam Sare of Southchurch in Essex heard 'the cries and groans' of Alice Southcherche's (unnamed) mother 'labouring in childbirth' on 1 November 1304 and recalled this in 1329, and John Barnard heard Alice Brugge crying out as she gave birth to her daughter Isabel in Haresfield, Gloucestershire on 13 August 1423. Margery Sumpter gave birth to her daughter Christine in Colchester, Essex early in the morning of 13 August 1411, and fifteen years later William Saundre recalled that he had heard her 'labour and cry out' during the night.[14]

Midwives

The word 'midwife', spelt *mid(d)ewyf* in Middle English, derives from the Old English words for 'with' and 'woman'. As documents in medieval England were often written in French, the word *sage femme*, literally 'wise woman', was also often used, and in modern French, *sage-femme* still means 'midwife'. In the early 1380s, the 'common midwife' of the Norfolk village of Braydeston was Cecily Goodfellow. Margaret Webbe and Margery Kellehog worked as midwives in Essex in the 1330s and 1340s, Magota Payn worked in Derby in the 1380s, Christine Ichene worked in Hampshire in the 1380s, and Isabel Harper worked in Yorkshire in the 1420s.[15] The register of John of Gaunt, Duke of Lancaster, reveals that a woman named Elyot or Ilote worked as a *middewyf* in Leicester. In early June 1372, John summoned Ilote ninety miles to Hertford Castle, lending her a cart and cart-driver to speed her journey, to assist his second wife Constanza of Castile either when she gave birth to their daughter Catalina of Lancaster or during her pregnancy.[16] Leicester was one of Duke John's towns, and it is likely that Ilote had aided at the birth of one or several of John's older children and that he trusted her.

Pernell St Omer laboured night and day with her daughter Alice, born in Wiltshire on 25 March 1340. Joan Mertok, a servant of Pernell's father-in-law, and Alice Kyngesmulle helped her through the difficult birth. During John Worthe's birth in Little Horsted in Sussex in early 1356, local resident John Scharp, aged about twenty-two, 'fetched a woman called Maud Swaneslone to act as *midewyf*'. Agnes Trim was in bed with her husband William at dawn on 8 March 1390, in Dauntsey, Wiltshire, when a man called Thomas Taberwell came to the door and asked her to be midwife to Elizabeth Daundesey, in labour with her son Walter. Nicholas Gryffon was born in Brixworth, Northamptonshire on 5 June 1426, and his father John sent a servant called William Selysby to fetch the midwife; it was raining, and William, in his haste, slipped on the wet path and broke his knee and ankle. Isabel Harper was the midwife when Joan Lely was born in Drax, Yorkshire on 12 October 1424, and 'brought a comb for Joan as soon as she saw her born, because she had a hairy head'. When Isabel Mare gave birth to her son Giles in Mears Ashby, Northamptonshire on 5 December 1307, Maud Faber was one of the women who helped her during labour. Maud had a thirty-seven-year-old son, so must have been in her fifties or older.[17]

Multiple Births

Edward I and Leonor of Castile's youngest daughter Elizabeth of Rhuddlan, Countess of Hereford (b. 1282), gave birth to twin boys around 1309 or 1312. Edward de Bohun was the elder twin and drowned in Scotland in 1334, and William (d. 1360), Earl of Northampton and a great-grandfather of Henry V, was the younger. As an abbey cartulary

Pregnancy and Childbirth (2)

specifically noted that the brothers were twins (*duo gemelli nobiles, Edwardus et Willielmus*), they were perhaps identical.[18] The twins' mother survived the birth, though died after bearing their sister Isabella in 1316. When Agnes Sancta Cruce, a landowner in Nottinghamshire, died in 1301, her heirs were her five daughters: Joan, twenty-four; Margery, twenty-two; Elizabeth, twenty-one; and twins Cecily and Margaret, much younger than their sisters and only five years old. Laurence and Philip Pavely were twins born on c. 15 August 1257, and when their father Robert died in March 1288, Laurence, as the elder twin, was his sole heir. Juliana Sompnour bore twin boys, Henry and John, in Weathersfield, Essex on 12 March 1351; Henry died at age ten, but John lived into adulthood. Werburga Prestcote gave birth to twin boys in Devon on 18 January 1403, and sadly if not entirely surprisingly, 'died instantly after their birth'. John Warde's wife, whose name was not recorded, bore twin sons in London on 2 February 1405 and apparently survived, and on 4 December 1423, Edith Martyn gave birth to her sons Vincent and Laurence in Woodsford, Dorset. It seems that they all lived. Juliana Portman gave birth to twin boys, Thomas and John, in Buxlow, Suffolk on 4 October 1274, and they all survived; the twins were still alive twenty-three years later. Finally, in 1369 the twins Beatrice Rayner and Maud Croxton, aged forty-six, were named as co-heirs to their underage great-nephew John Gaunt in Middlesex, with their fifty-year-old unmarried sister Christina Gaunt.[19]

Otherwise, there is little direct evidence for multiple births in late medieval England, and sometimes we can only postulate that siblings might have been twins because their stated ages were the same in inquisitions. One example is Elizabeth, Duchess of Norfolk, and her sister Joan, Lady Abergavenny, born c. the late 1360s. They and their younger sister Margaret were the heirs of their brother Thomas Fitzalan, Earl of Arundel, in 1415, and all the jurors who took part in Thomas's inquisition post mortem gave exactly the same ages for Elizabeth and Joan.[20] Another possible example is Richard Neville, Earl of Warwick (d. 1471), and his sister Cecily, Duchess of Warwick and Countess of Worcester (d. 1450). Cecily's date of birth is not known for certain, but Richard was born on 22 November 1428, and 22 November is the feast of St Cecilia. Furthermore, the siblings married on the same day, and if they were not twins, it is difficult to fit Cecily into the birth order of the Neville siblings.[21] Finally, Richard III's friend Francis, Viscount Lovell, born in 1456, was almost certainly a twin to his sister Joan, and they had a younger sister, Frideswide, as well.[22] At least some people in late medieval England appear to have believed that a woman who gave birth to twins must have had intercourse with two men.[23]

Mortality Rates in Childbirth and Infancy

A Caesarean birth was a last resort as it was always fatal for the mother, and probably more than 10% of all births were stillbirths. The percentage of all confinements in the Middle Ages and the sixteenth century which resulted in the mother's death has been estimated at 2%, or one in fifty.[24] As Ian Mortimer states, this perhaps does not look too horrendous at first glance, but given that most married women gave birth more than once and some bore more than a dozen children, every pregnancy was 'like a game of Russian Roulette, played with a fifty-barrel gun'. Giving birth a dozen times was akin to firing that gun a dozen times.[25]

For a woman labouring in vain to bring forth an infant who had already died inside her, the *Trotula* recommended that she lie on a linen sheet and that four strong men each pulled at a corner, which would cause the woman to give birth immediately. The authors were aware that some women tear while giving birth, and recommended sewing the rupture in the perineum 'in three or four places with silk thread' and healing the wound with comfrey.[26] Another medieval medical text was the *Sekenesse of Wymmen*, 'Sickness of Women', a fifteenth-century translation of several chapters of a thirteenth-century work by Gilbertus Anglicus called *Compendium Medicinae*. Perhaps surprisingly, this work demonstrated more concern for women enduring a difficult labour than for the child: 'for whan the womman is fieble and the chield may nat come oute, than it is better that the chield be slayne than the moder of the chield die'.[27]

The infant mortality rate was also horrific, and as many as one in six children did not live to see their first birthday.[28] Even privilege and wealth made little difference. Three of Edward III and Queen Philippa's twelve children – two of their seven sons and one of their five daughters – died at a few days or weeks old; three more of their daughters died as teenagers, and only four of the royal children outlived the king. Of the at least fourteen and perhaps sixteen children born to Leonor of Castile and Edward I, Leonor outlived all but six and Edward outlived all but

Pregnancy and Childbirth (2)

four of them. At least five and perhaps seven of their children died when they were under two years old, and three others died at the ages of five, six and ten. Edward and Leonor's daughter Elizabeth of Rhuddlan, second youngest of the royal offspring, died shortly after giving birth to her tenth child in May 1316, after surviving the birth of twins a few years earlier; she was thirty-three. Two of Elizabeth's four older sisters who survived childhood, Eleanor of Windsor and Joan of Acre, died at the ages of twenty-nine and thirty-five respectively, and although it is not known for certain what killed them, given their ages and the pattern of their childbearing, it seems possible that their deaths were connected to pregnancy or childbirth.

On the other hand, Joan of Acre's eldest daughter Eleanor, Lady Despenser (b. 1292), gave birth to at least eleven children between c. 1308 and c. 1330, and ten of them survived childhood. Twelve children of Roger Mortimer, first Earl of March (1287–1330) and Joan Geneville (b. 1286) lived into adulthood, and Joan herself died in 1356 at age seventy. Elizabeth of Rhuddlan's daughter Margaret de Bohun, Countess of Devon (b. 1311), gave birth to sixteen or seventeen children and died in 1391 at eighty years old, and Edward III's granddaughter Joan Beaufort, Countess of Westmorland, had about sixteen children and died in 1440 in her early or mid-sixties. Between the 1430s and late 1450s, Jacquetta of Luxembourg, dowager Duchess of Bedford, gave birth to fourteen or fifteen children during her second marriage to Sir Richard Woodville, of whom twelve lived into adulthood. Jacquetta herself lived until 1472, aged at least fifty-five.

In June 1282, late in her pregnancy, Margery Torkard of Stapleford on the Derbyshire/Nottinghamshire border suffered from 'great weakness', and gave birth to a son 'scarcely 6 thumbs in length'. The little boy lived long enough to be baptised, but then died.[29] Joan Otringdene or Oteringdenne married George Lavertone at Otterden in Kent on Wednesday, 31 December 1292. Joan became pregnant immediately: she gave birth to their daughter, also Joan, at dawn on Monday, 28 September 1293, but died very soon afterwards. Andrew, rector of Otterden, gave her the last rites, and baptised little Joan Lavertone 'in her mother's chamber ... alive and crying'. There was just enough time for the infant's godfather and two godmothers, John Wynefeld, Eleanor Sindisham and Aubrey Stonacre, to arrive for the ceremony, but little Joan 'lived until sunrise of the same day and then died'.[30] In June 1374 in the Lincolnshire village of Whaplode, Joan, wife of twenty-two-year-old John Vesy, was heavily pregnant. John recalled twenty-two years later that Joan 'died pregnant of a son, Christopher'. The boy survived and was still alive in 1396.[31] This surely reveals that Joan died before she gave birth and that midwives removed her son from her womb after death. At Christmas 1346, Agnes, wife of John Clerk, died in Stortford, Hertfordshire, while she was pregnant. John was forty at the time, though Agnes's age is not recorded.[32] Unfortunately, in this case, Agnes's infant died with her.

Robert Abbot of Stapleford died on the day he was born and baptised, 12 November 1307, and Robert Colbrooke died in infancy in Pinhoe, Devon around six a.m. on 3 May 1400. His father Nicholas went to the parish church to summon the local parson to come to his house and perform Robert's obsequies.[33] Alice Partryg or Partrich died after giving birth in Salisbury on 6 October 1411, and the infant died too. Her husband Richard, who was at least forty-five at the time, reflected bitterly many years later that 'lack of good care' killed his wife and child.[34] Thomas Russell of Gloucestershire died in 1431 leaving his widow Joan pregnant, and some months later she gave birth to a daughter, Margery, who died at two days old.[35] When Margaret Bonevyle was in labour with her son William in Shute, Devon on 31 August 1392, several village residents heard her screaming out to the Virgin Mary for help, and rushed to the local church to pray for her. Margaret survived the difficult birth, and her son lived into adulthood and became the ward of Richard 'Dick' Whittington, mayor of London.[36]

Chapter 11

Pregnancy and Childbirth (3)

Baptism and Godparents

Infants were baptised in their local church or chapel on the day of their birth or the following day, and the ceremony was called 'making the infant a Christian' while taking part in the baptism as a godparent was called 'raising the infant from the sacred font'. Nicholaa Neville was born in Blaxwell, Wiltshire on Wednesday, 29 May 1297, and was baptised in the church of Whiteparish the next day; Hugh Plessetis was born in Kidlington, Oxfordshire around six a.m. on 25 April 1295, and was baptised by the abbot of Osney in the local church around nine a.m. the following day. Beatrice Hastang was born in Quinton, Northamptonshire in the morning of 20 July 1309 and was baptised at Vespers or sunset on the same day.[1] Elizabeth Staundon, however, born in London on 21 January 1405, was not baptised until 2 February, the feast of the Purification. An inquisition of 26 July 1426 declared that Elizabeth had turned twenty-one on 2 February that year, on the date of her baptism rather than her date of birth.[2] Joan Haym was born in Southam, Gloucestershire on 9 August 1357, and was baptised in the local parish church on the same day; her godparents were Joan Alvard, Amflesia Mareschall and John Taillour. The unnamed chaplain who baptised her must have been in a foul mood, as for some unexplained reason he struck forty-two-year-old John atte Halle, one of the people present in the church, with a stick and 'broke his head' (thankfully John survived, and recalled this assault eighteen years later). After Nicholas, son and heir of John and Christine atte Hull, was baptised in Ashbrittle, Somerset on 4 May 1368, his father asked the parson to write the words 'Nycol the sone of John atte Hull and Crystyne his wife was y bore' in the church missal.[3]

Boys had two godfathers and one godmother, and girls had two godmothers and one godfather. They had to be chosen carefully, as acting as a person's godparent created a spiritual affinity between the two families which required a dispensation from the pope if the families wished to intermarry in the future. William Welde of Dinnington in Somerset, aged about twenty-six, 'flatly refused' Thomas Chasteleyn's invitation to be the godfather of Thomas's newborn daughter Joan in March 1348 'because it was possible that he might survive the said Thomas and marry Isabel, the latter's wife' (one assumes that William kept the real reason to himself rather than telling Thomas to his face that he hoped to marry his widow one day). Richard Alisaundre of Northamptonshire, aged about thirty-five, turned down the invitation to be Agnes Burnby's godfather in 1356 on the rather creepy grounds that he might wish to marry the infant in the future.[4] Pope Clement VI issued a dispensation in 1351 for Thomas Lench and his wife Alice Boteler, who had married even though Thomas was the godfather of Alice's son from a previous marriage. Thomas proffered the excuse, a most unflattering one for Alice, that he 'knew no-one else whom he could marry at the time of the pestilence', i.e. the great pandemic of the Black Death in 1348/49.[5] In 1431 in Exeter, Richard Mounfort and his second wife Joan Schether failed to realise that, as Richard's first wife Ebote was godmother to Joan's child from a previous marriage, this created a spiritual impediment to their own marriage. Alice Brank's first husband John Gilberne had stood as godfather to her second husband John Brank's illegitimate daughter, which required a dispensation in 1437 after Alice and Brank already had several children together.[6]

Infants were often named after a godparent, such as Joan Haym, above, named after her godmother Joan Alvard. In January 1362, Robert de Vere (d. 1392), future Earl of Oxford and Duke of Ireland, and the beloved of Richard II, was named after his godfather and maternal great-uncle Robert Ufford, Earl of Suffolk (1298–1369). De Vere's other godfather was Simon Sudbury, then Bishop of London and later Archbishop of Canterbury, beheaded outside the Tower of London during the Great Uprising (or Peasants' Revolt) in June 1381, and his godmother was Alice, widow of Sir Andrew Bures.[7] Sir Ralph Basset, Lord of Weldon Basset in Northamptonshire, angrily punched his servant Richard Reve on the neck during the baptism of John Aylesbury on 6 May 1334, after Reve asked him why little John was not named after Basset or his other godfather Sir Warin Latimer.[8]

Sometimes a child was named for the saint on whose feast day s/he was born instead. Anne Cheyne was born in Westbury, Wiltshire on 26 July 1428, and an attendee at her baptism 'heard Anne's godmothers arguing about Anne's name in the church, and they agreed to name her Anne because she was born on the feast of that saint'.[9] This indicates that at least sometimes, it was godparents rather than parents who chose an infant's name. On 26 December 1357 at William Deyncourt's baptism in Leicestershire, his godfathers Sir Roger Belers and Thomas, abbot of Croxton, argued 'as to which of them had named him first', until finally, they agreed to call him William instead, 'as most of his ancestors were named'.[10] Infants were also sometimes named after a saint favoured by their parents, such as Edmund Colville in 1288, whose father Roger had travelled to the shrine of St Edmund of Pontigny in France. At the baptism of Katherine Hildeyerd in Holderness in March 1322, people in the church wondered why she was not named after one of her godmothers, Beatrice Coleville or Christiana Ligard, and learned that 'for love of St Katherine she was so named'.[11] In other cases, children were named after a parent, grandparent, aunt or uncle, and confusingly, the same first name was sometimes given to a younger sibling. Sir John Grey of Rotherfield (1300–59) had three sons and named two of them John, and the Londoner John Tettysbury or Tiddesbury had two daughters, Joan and Joan, born in c. 1382 and c. 1391.[12] The two eldest sons of John Paston of East Anglia (1421–66), born in 1442 and 1444, were both named John.

Infants, wrapped in swaddling clothes, were carried to their baptism by their nurse or godmother, because the mother, who had not yet been purified after the birth and was still recovering, did not attend the baptism. Four or six men each carried an unlit torch or candle to the church with the child, and when s/he returned home afterwards, the torches were lit. At the baptism of Joan Argentein in Halesworth, Suffolk in June 1413, four men holding lit torches stood around the font as she was baptised. Robert atte Chirche was dressed in 'a linen cloth called *crisme* marked with a cross of red and gold silk' during his baptism in Epping, Essex in February 1375. Christine Ichene was the midwife who aided at the birth of Richard Inkepenne in Woolston, Hampshire on 14 August 1389, and carried him in a boat across the River Itchen for his baptism.[13] When the infant was of noble birth, a considerable amount of ceremony took place. The Anglo-Scottish noblewoman Philippa Strathbogie was born in Gainsborough, Lincolnshire on 21 March 1362, and Simon Curtays and three other clerks carried a 'red carpet over her on four lances' as she was carried into All Saints Church for her baptism the same day. John Mowbray, second son and ultimate heir of Thomas Mowbray, Earl of Nottingham and later Duke of Norfolk, was born in Calais on 3 August 1390, and baptised there on 9 August (and was therefore deemed to have turned twenty-one on 9 August 1411). All the knights, squires, gentlemen and aldermen of Calais accompanied the infant in a procession to the church, and after John's baptism, he was taken back to his father's house with four knights and squires carrying a 'golden awning' above him and with one of the earl's squires carrying a 'sword erect' behind him.[14] Infants were almost always given gifts by their godparents during their baptism, and a 'little silver bell' features frequently, as do silver plates and goblets, and purses with cash. Robert Stodhowe of Yorkshire was given a 'red cow' by his godfather, the vicar of East Cowton, in April 1383. In his will of 1390, the armourer William Trippelowe left 3s 4d to 'each of his children in Christ, viz., *godchilders*'.[15]

Churches were very busy places, and baptisms often took place in the same church and at the same time as weddings or funerals. As also sometimes happened at weddings, when wealthier people attended baptisms, they scattered coins to be gathered by the poor. At the baptism of John Aylesbury in Northamptonshire in May 1334, John's godparents Sir Warin Latimer and Sir Ralph Basset and his wife Joan 'threw pence everywhere'. Geoffrey Julian, aged twenty-seven, managed to collect 80d of it. When Richard Redman was baptised in Harewood, Yorkshire on 18 October 1406, a servant of his parents named Thomas Warde 'carried two silver platters to the church, holding gold and silver for throwing to bystanders'.[16] It was the custom for the godparents and other attendees to drink sweet red wine and eat bread once the baptism was over. After Elizabeth Briene was baptised in the church of St Peter, Paul's Wharf in London on 13 March 1381, her father Guy had a servant bring 'some pots full of wine called *bastard* to the church', and Richard Berners provided three 'hot loaves' at the baptism of his daughter Margery in West Horsley, Surrey on 30 November 1408. Thomas Wyntereshull's father provided a gallon of sweet wine for his godparents and other attendees at his baptism in Worplesdon, Surrey in October 1392.[17] The wine was drunk out of silver-gilt goblets and jugs wherever the parents' financial means permitted it.[18] After the baptism of Robert Todenham in

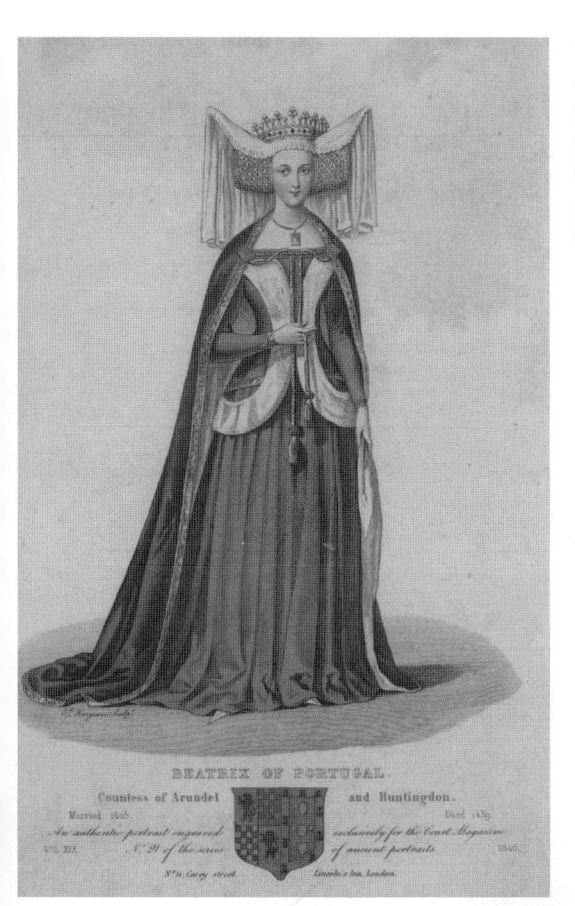

Beatriz of Portugal, countess of Arundel, Surrey and Huntingdon (*c.* 1380/82-1439); a nineteenth-century image of her effigy in the Fitzalan Chapel of Arundel Castle, Sussex, showing her wide, horned headdress. (Public domain)

Isabel of Portugal, duchess of Burgundy (1397-1471), Beatriz's half-sister and a granddaughter of John of Gaunt, duke of Lancaster; she wears an elaborate heart-shaped bourrelet. (Public domain)

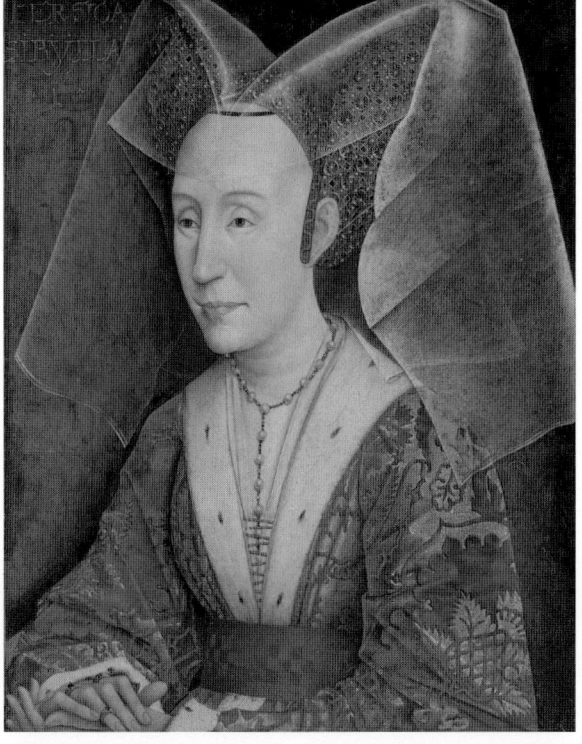

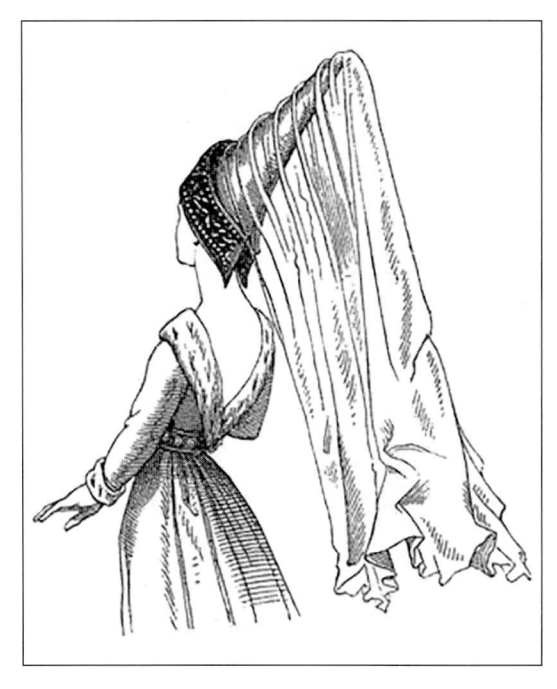

Left: A fifteenth-century hennin. (Public domain)

Below left: A nineteenth-century image of the effigies of Edward III (d. 1377) and his queen Philippa of Hainault (d. 1369) in Westminster Abbey. Philippa wears a tight *cotehardie* laced up the front and with buttoned sleeves, and a narrow hip-belt; her hair is encased in stiff net-like bags. (Public domain)

Below right: A nineteenth-century image of Edward III and Queen Philippa's son Lionel of Antwerp, duke of Clarence (1338-68), from a statuette on their tomb. Lionel, who married in 1342 at the age of 3, wears hose, a buttoned tunic with a hip-belt, and a cloak. (Public domain)

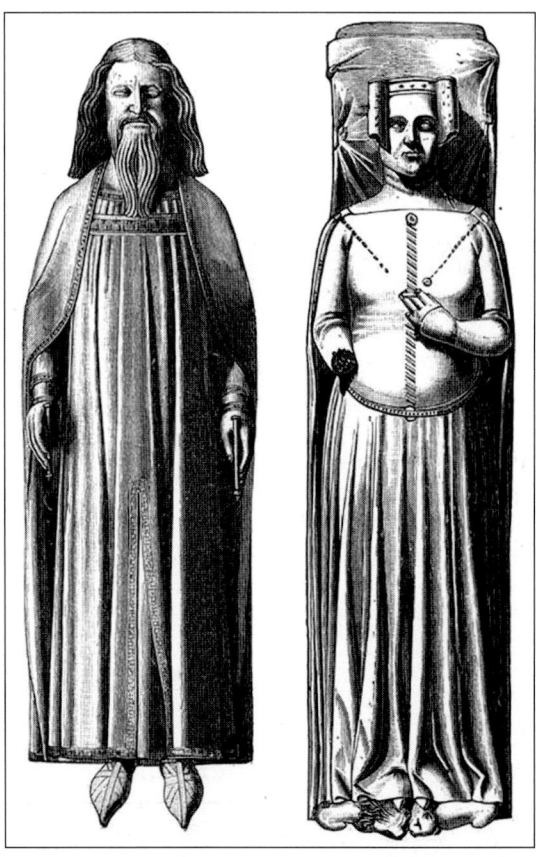

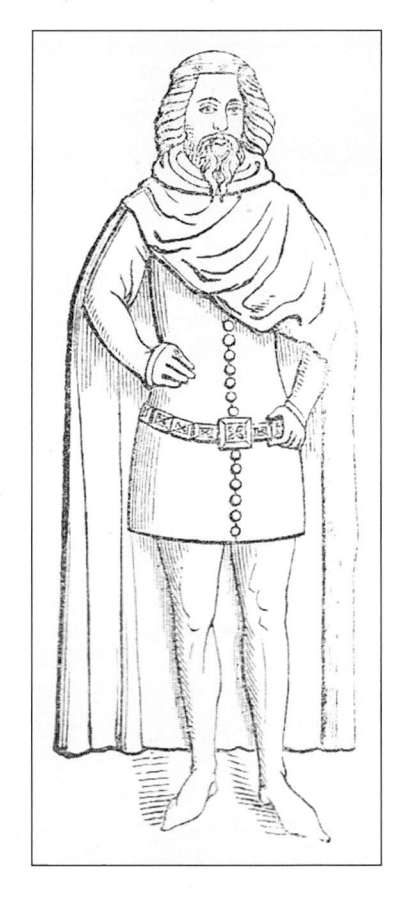

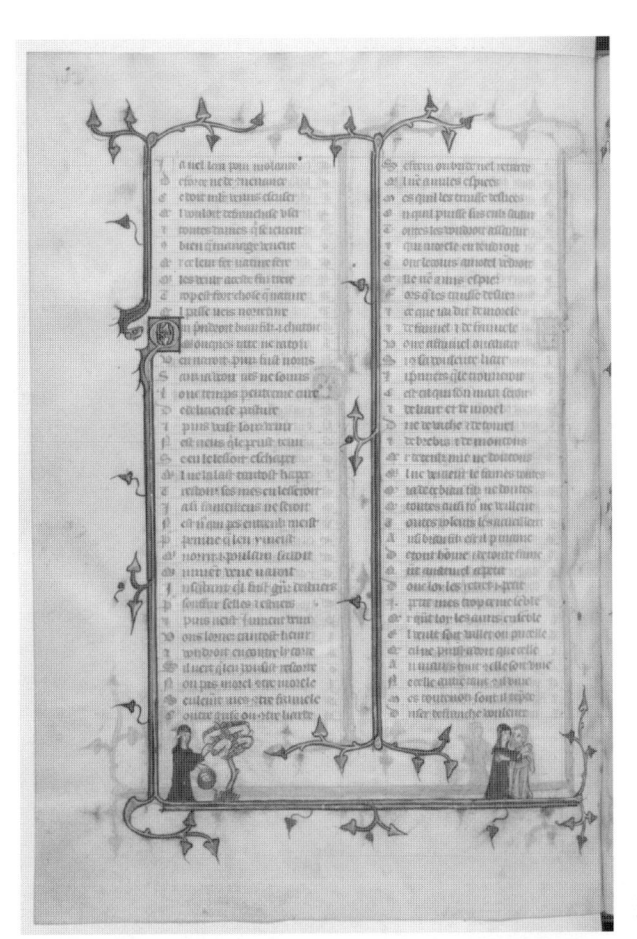

Right and below: An illustration from a fourteenth-century manuscript of the *Roman de la Rose*: a nun picks penises from a phallus tree. (Paris, Bibliothèque Nationale de France, MS. Fr. 25526, fo. 106v; public domain)

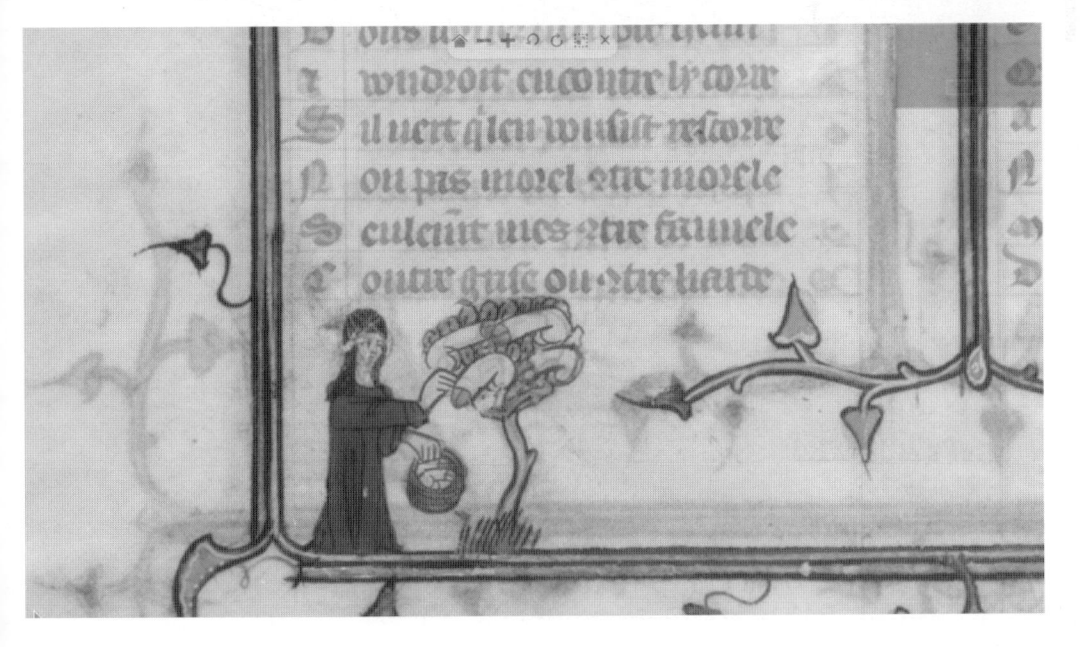

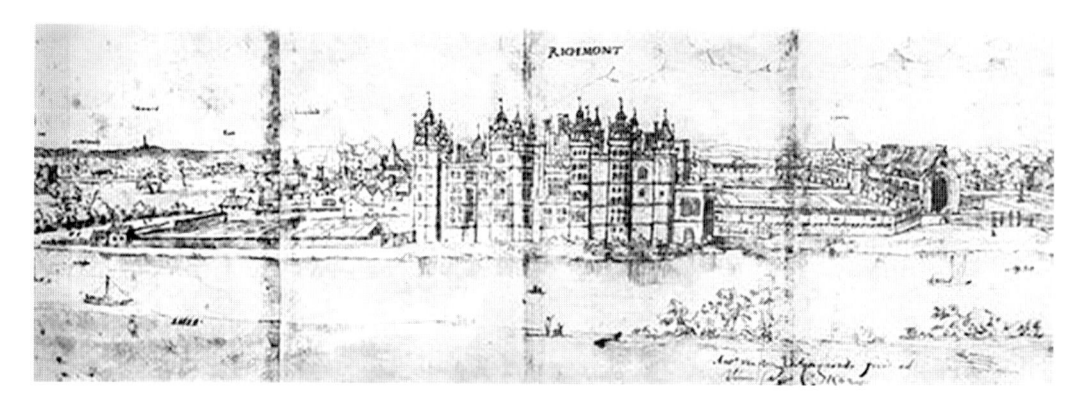

The palace of Sheen west of London, later Richmond Palace. Henry V had it rebuilt after it was pulled down on a devastated Richard II's orders in 1395, because his beloved wife Anne of Bohemia had died there ten months earlier. (Public domain)

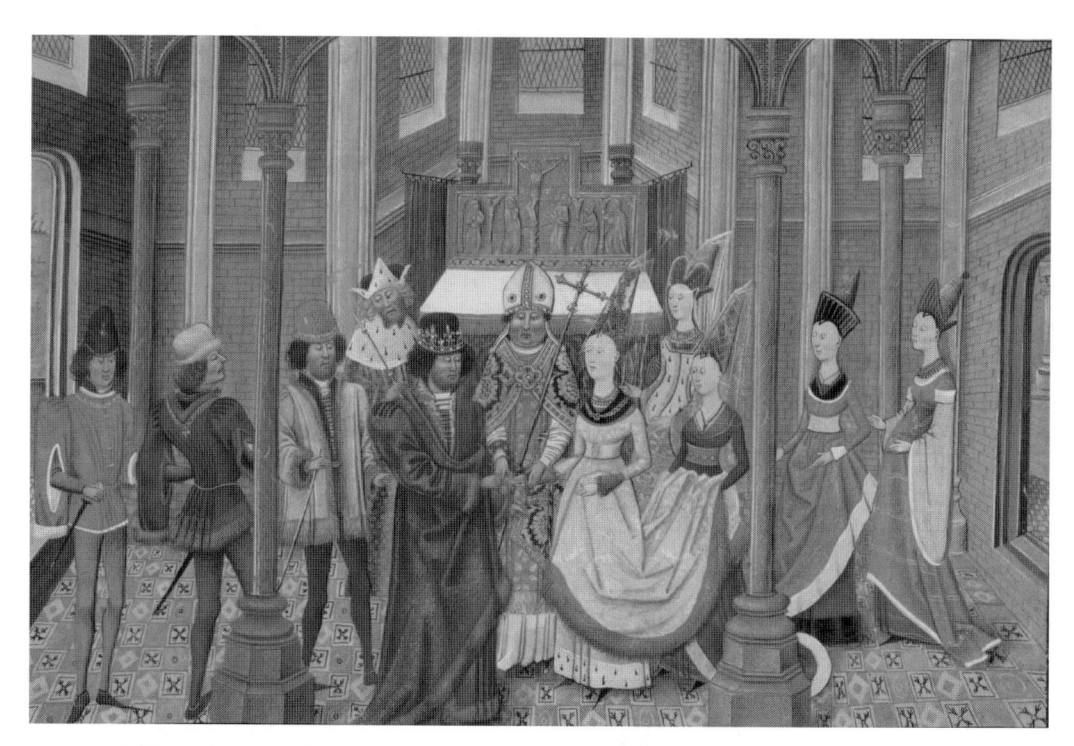

A fifteenth-century illustration of the wedding of King João of Portugal and Philippa of Lancaster in Porto in February 1387. (Jean Wavrin's *Chronique de France et d'Angleterre*; public domain)

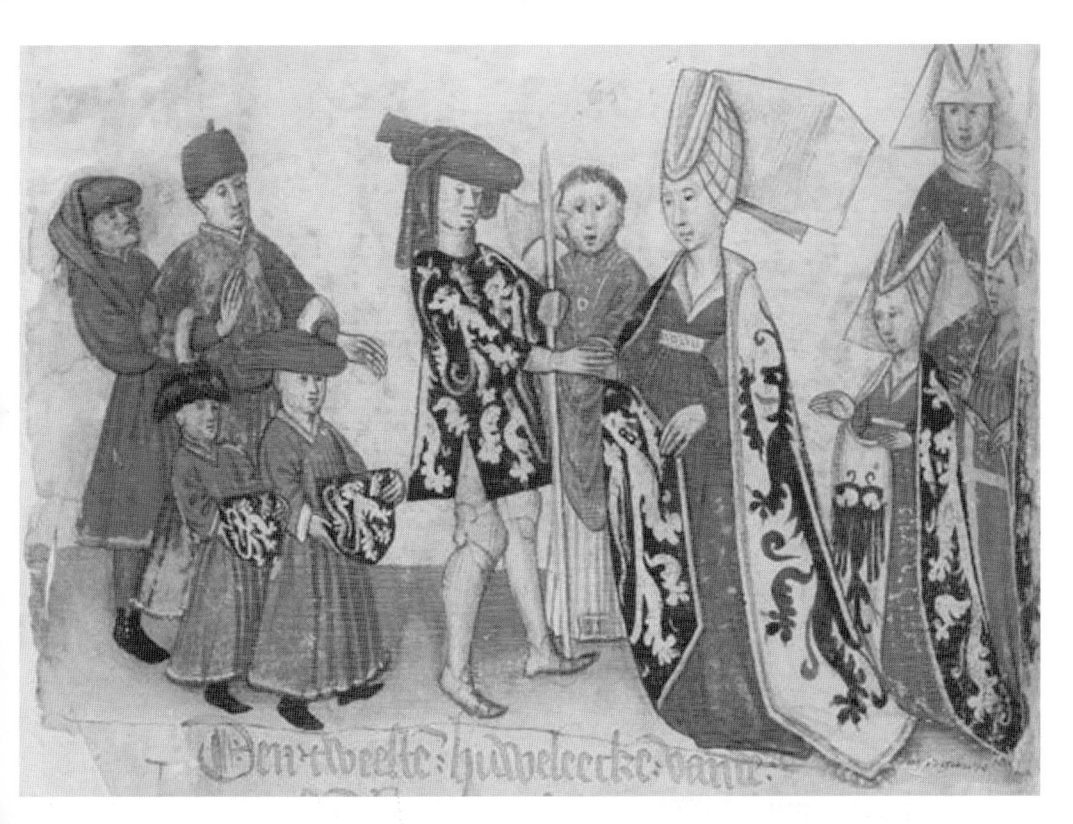

The wedding of Duke Jan I of Brabant (*c.* 1253-94), whose son Jan II (1275-1312) married Edward I of England's daughter Margaret in 1290, and his first wife Marguerite of France (1254-71), from the chronicle *Brabantsche Yeesten*. This manuscript of the chronicle dates to the fifteenth century, and the bridal pair's clothes are anachronistic. (Public domain)

The 1322 wedding of Charles IV of France (r. 1322-28), brother-in-law of Edward II of England, and his second wife Marie of Luxembourg (d. 1324), whose brother John 'the Blind', king of Bohemia, was killed fighting against Edward III at the battle of Crécy in 1346. (From *Les Grandes Chroniques de France*, Paris, Bibliothèque Nationale de France, MS. Fr. 2608, fo. 400r; public domain)

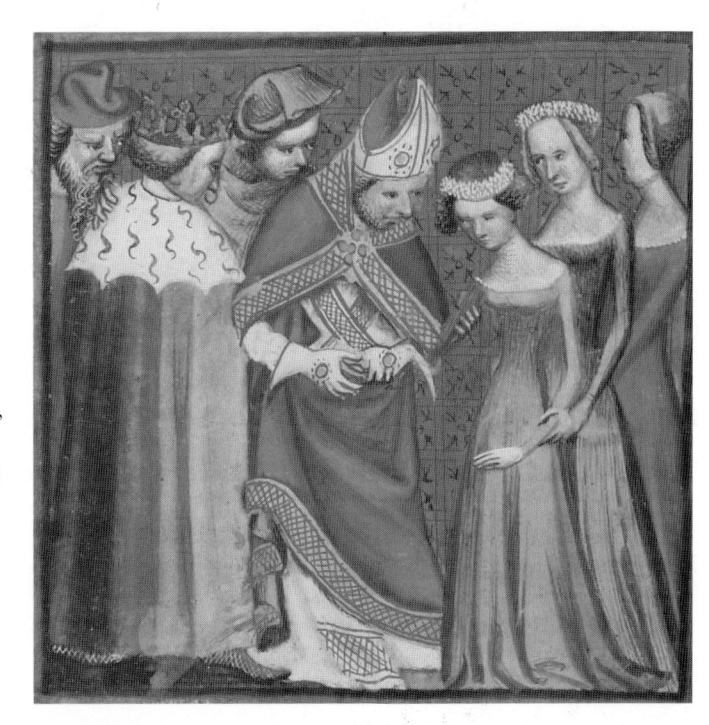

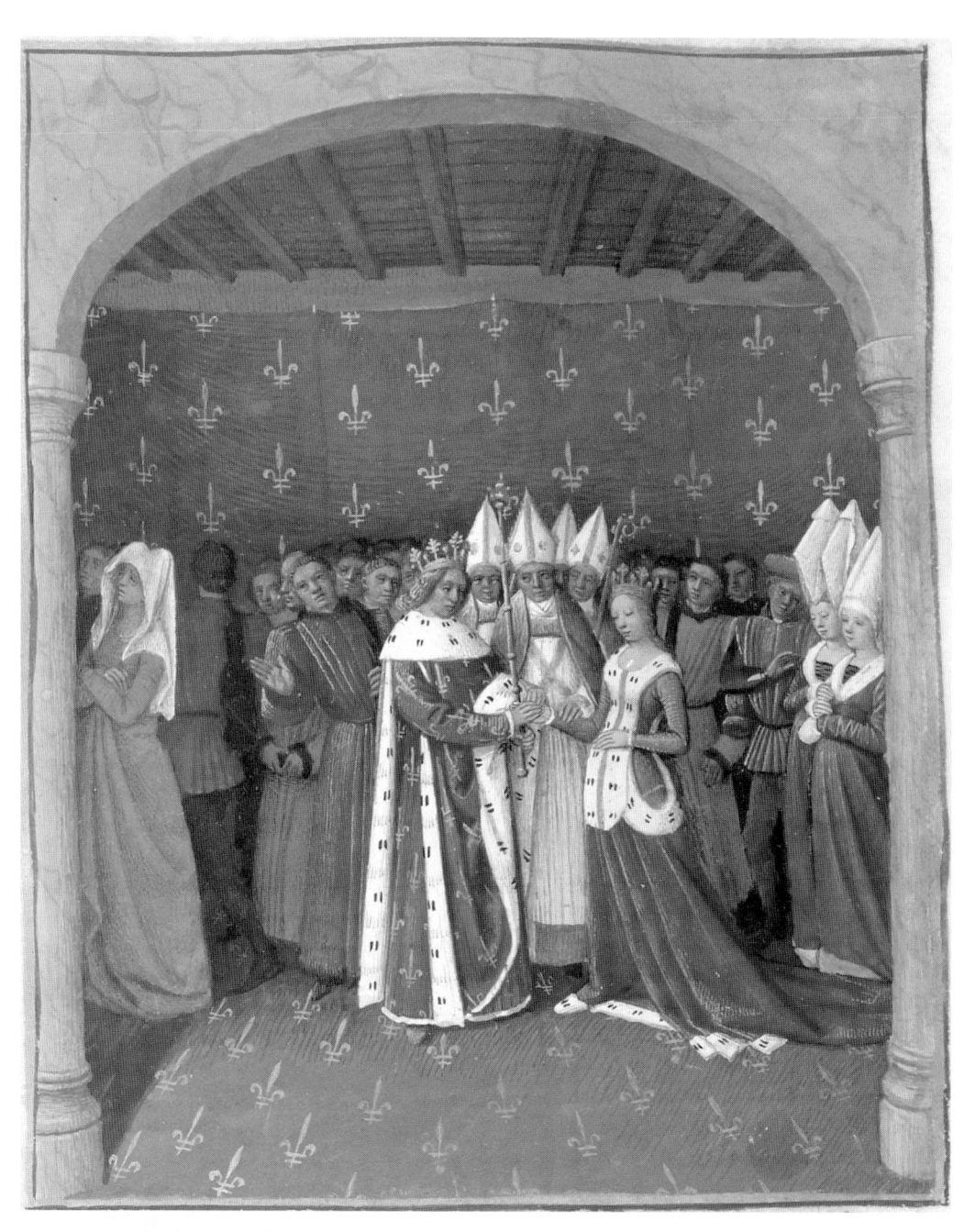

Another image of the wedding of Charles and Marie, who wears a fashionable sideless surcoat with fur, and whose unbound hair falls to her knees. On the left, Charles's first wife Blanche of Burgundy, imprisoned for adultery in 1314 and still alive in 1322, folds her arms and looks away. (From the Livre de Charles IV le Bel, Paris, BnF, MS. Fr. 6465, fo. 332; public domain)

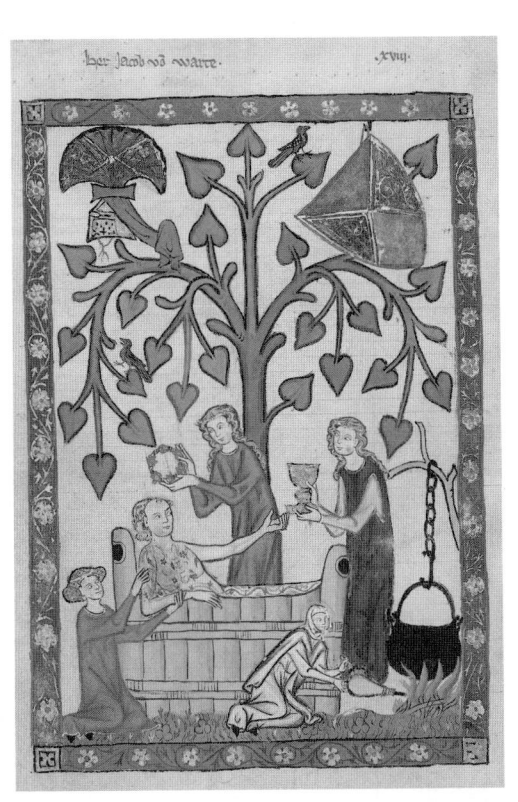

A medieval nobleman taking a bath in rose-water, *c.* 1305-40. (From the Codex Manesse, UB Heidelberg, Cod. Pal. germ. 848, fo. 46v; public domain)

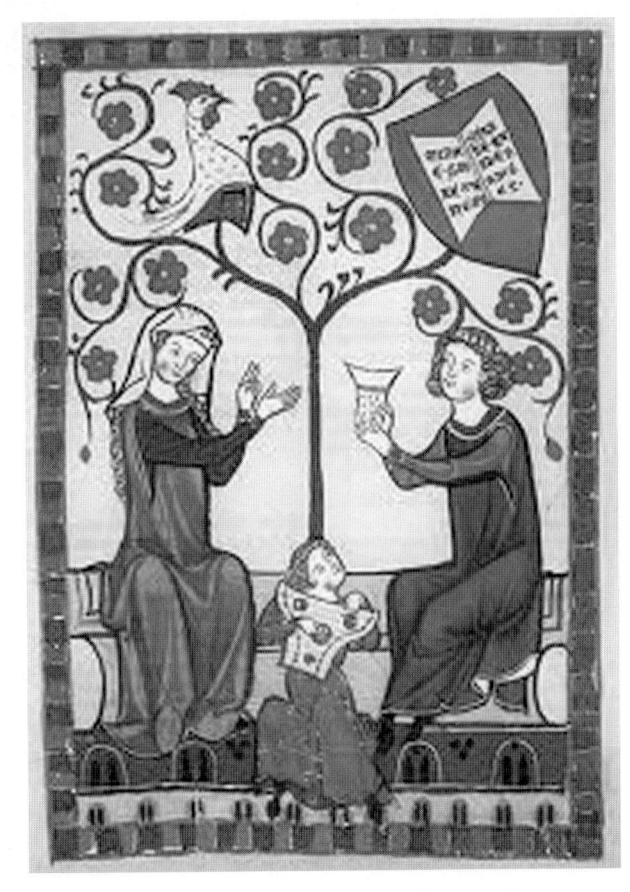

Medieval couples. (Codex Manesse)

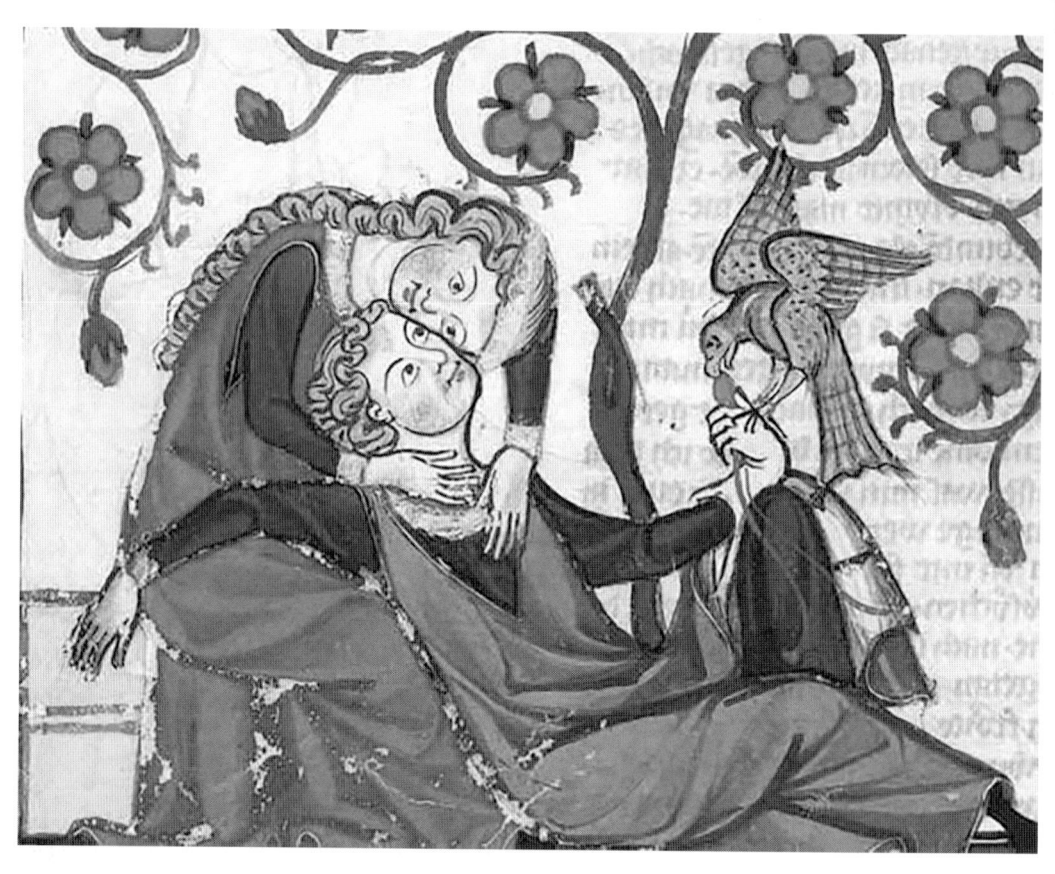

Above and left: Medieval couples. (Codex Manesse)

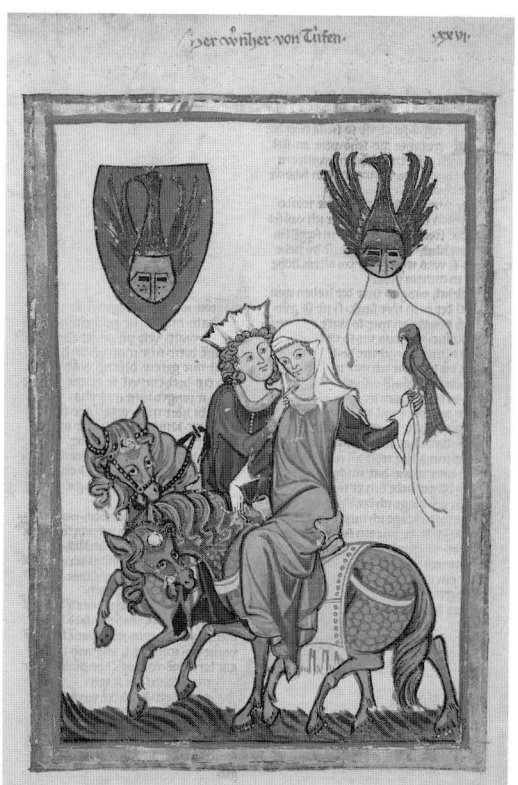

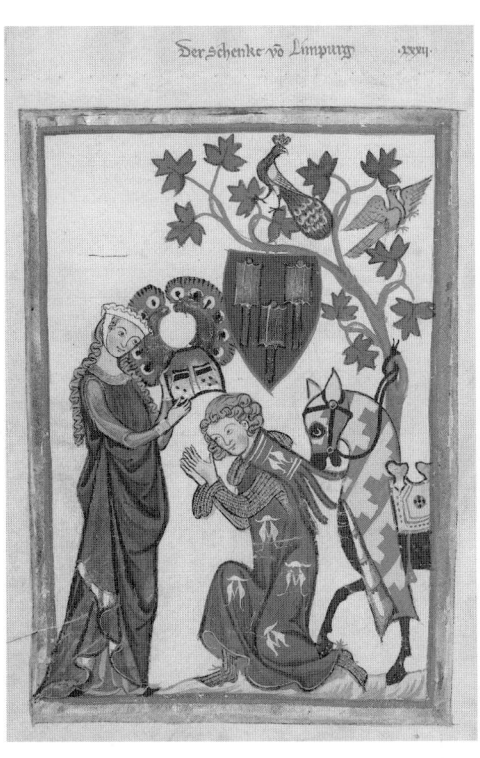

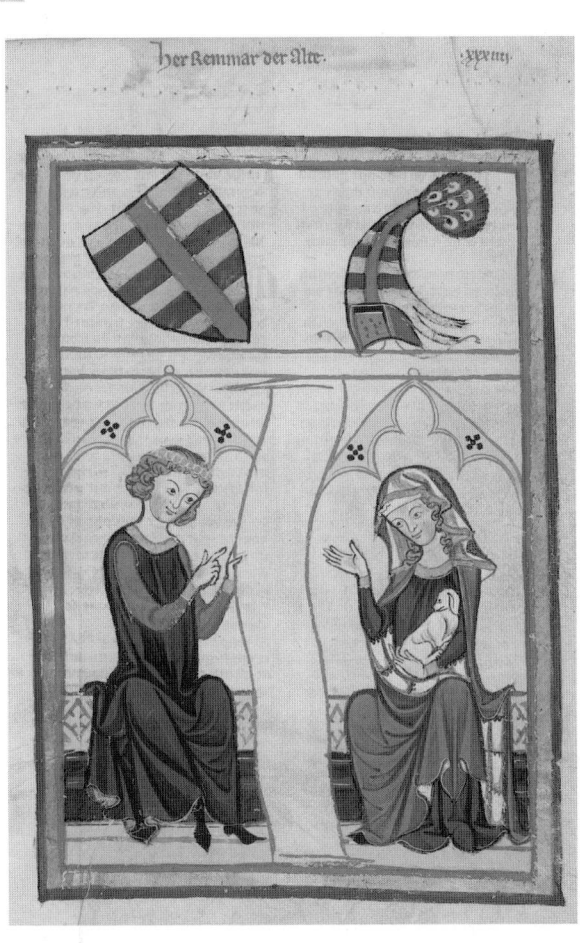

Medieval couples. (Codex Manesse)

Medieval couples. (Codex Manesse)

Medieval couples. (Codex Manesse)

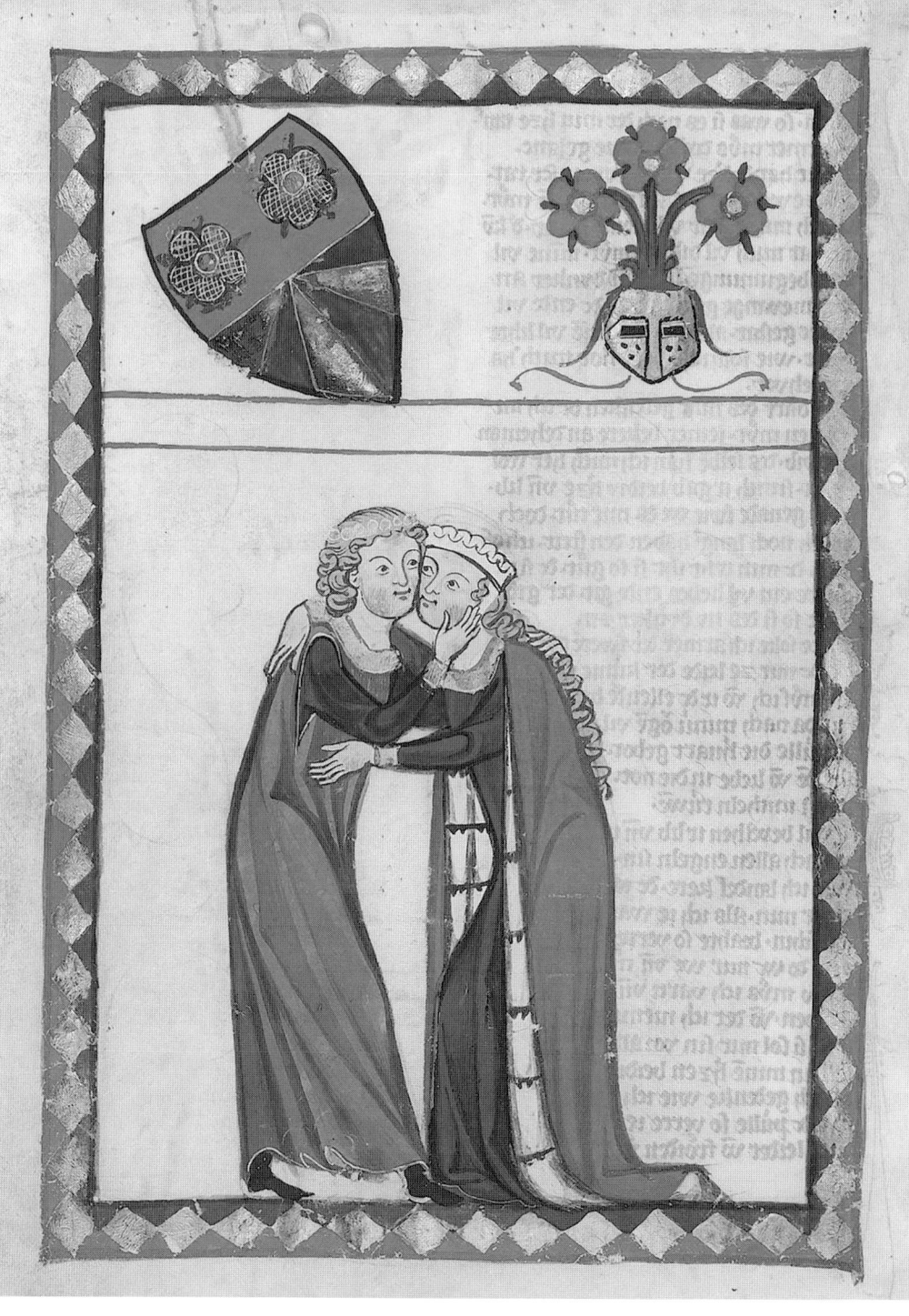

Right: A husband and wife taking a bath, *c*. 1350. (*Recueil de traités de médecine et image du monde,* Paris, BnF, MS. Fr. 12323, fo. 77r; public domain)

Below: A lady in a bathtub, being rescued by Lancelot; late thirteenth century. (From *Tristan en prose*, British Library Additional MS. 5474, fo. 144; made available under a Public Domain Mark)

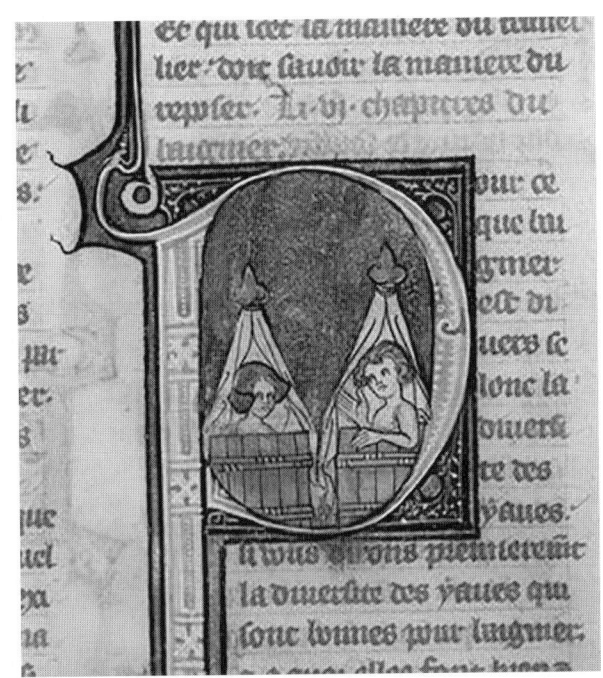

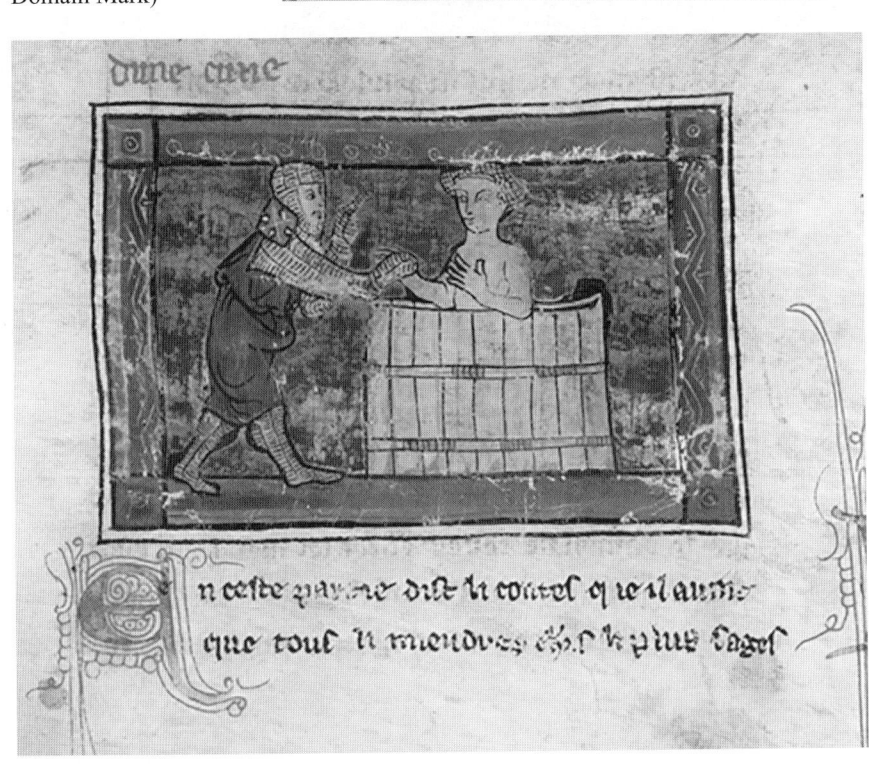

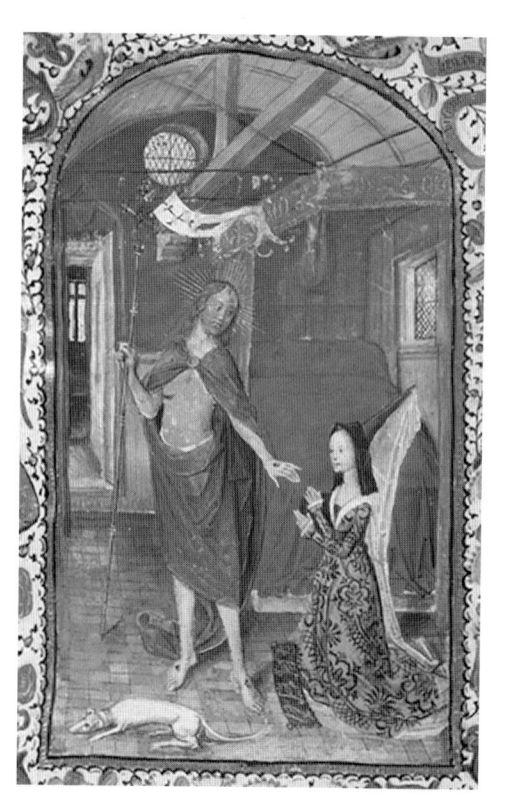

Margaret of York, duchess of Burgundy (1446-1503), kneeling in front of the resurrected Christ, wearing a hennin. (*Dialogue de la duchesse de Bourgogne a Jesus Christ*, British Library Additional MS. 7970, fo. 1v; made available under a Public Domain Mark)

The wedding of Jason and Creusa, and Medea taking her revenge; 1470s. (From the *Historie van Jason*, BL Additional MS. 10290, fo. 138; made available under a Public Domain Mark)

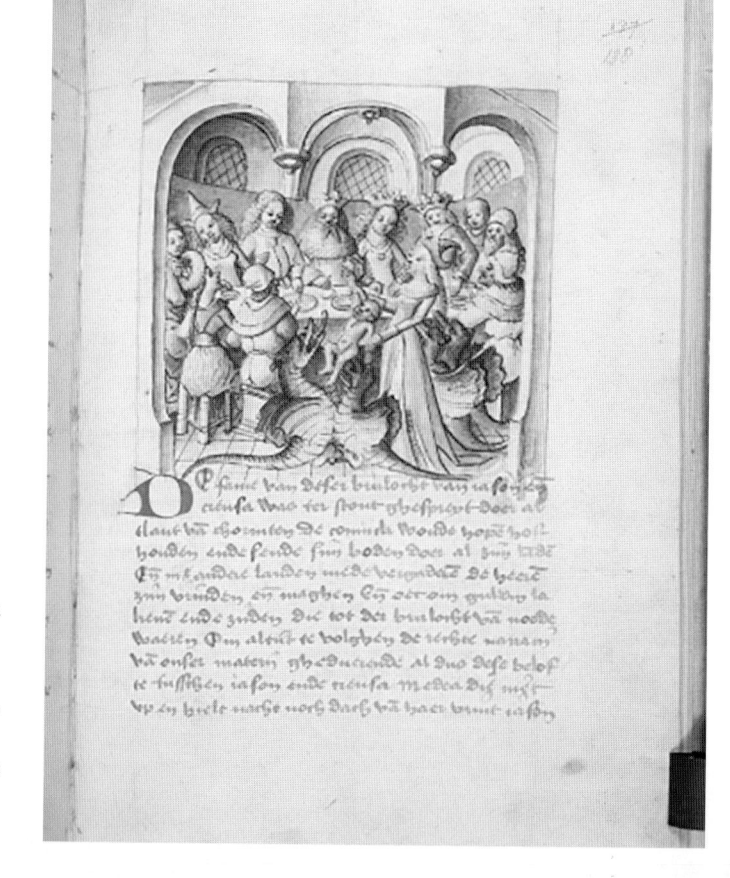

Right: Miniature of a crowned man and woman in bed, naked and embracing, with a dragon flying overhead; early fourteenth century. (From the *Roman d'Alexandre*, BL MS. Harley 4979, fo. 11; made available under a Public Domain Mark)

Below: The zodiac sign of Gemini presented as a naked couple; early fourteenth century. (From a fragmentary Book of Hours, BL Additional MS. 36684, fo. 6; made available under a Public Domain Mark)

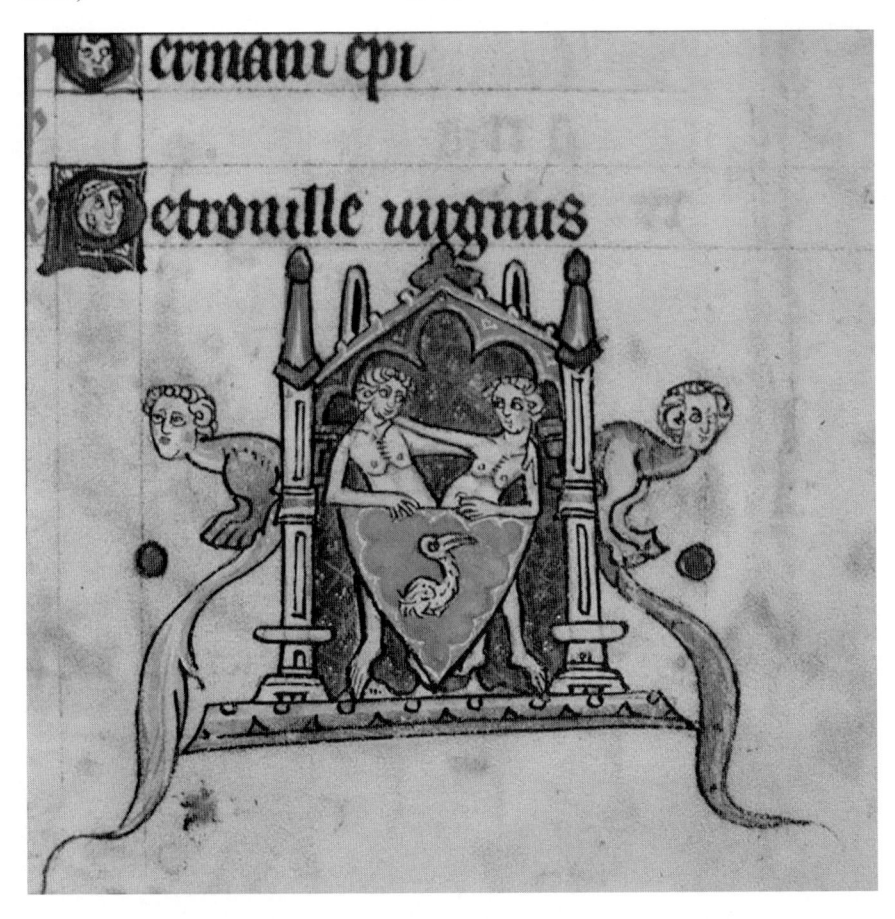

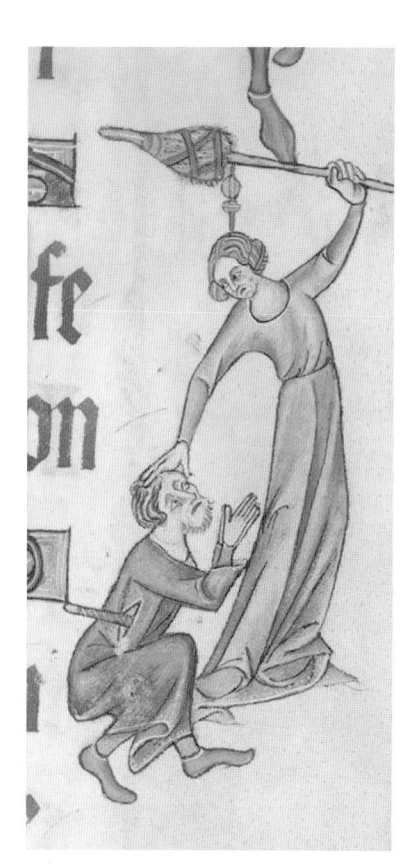

Left: A left-handed woman smiting an abject man with a broom, from the Luttrell Psalter, made for Sir Geoffrey Luttrell of Lincolnshire (d. 1345). (BL Additional MS. 42130, fo. 60; made available under a Public Domain Mark)

Below: Sir Geoffrey Luttrell in armour on horseback, with his wife Agnes Sutton and their daughter-in-law Beatrice Scrope. Both ladies wear a sheer veil held in place with a circlet, which leaves their hair uncovered on the top and sides of the head; a wimple covers their neck and chin. (BL Additional MS. 42130, fo. 202v; made available under a Public Domain Mark)

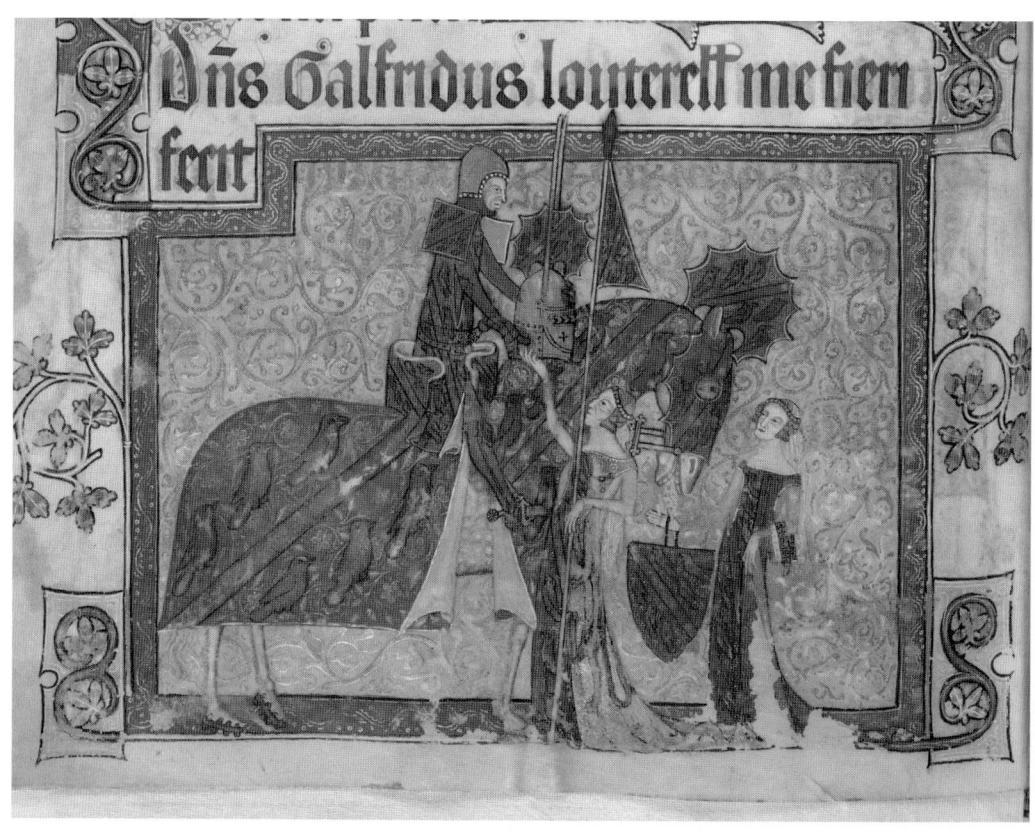

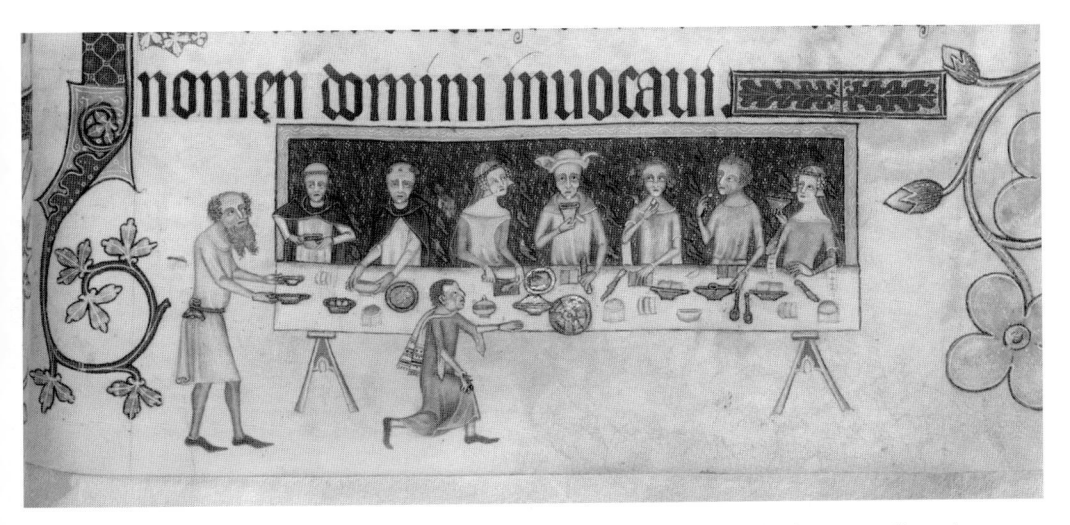

A feast from the Luttrell Psalter. Again, two of the women wear diaphanous veils and a circlet. (BL Additional MS. 42130, fo. 208; made available under a Public Domain Mark)

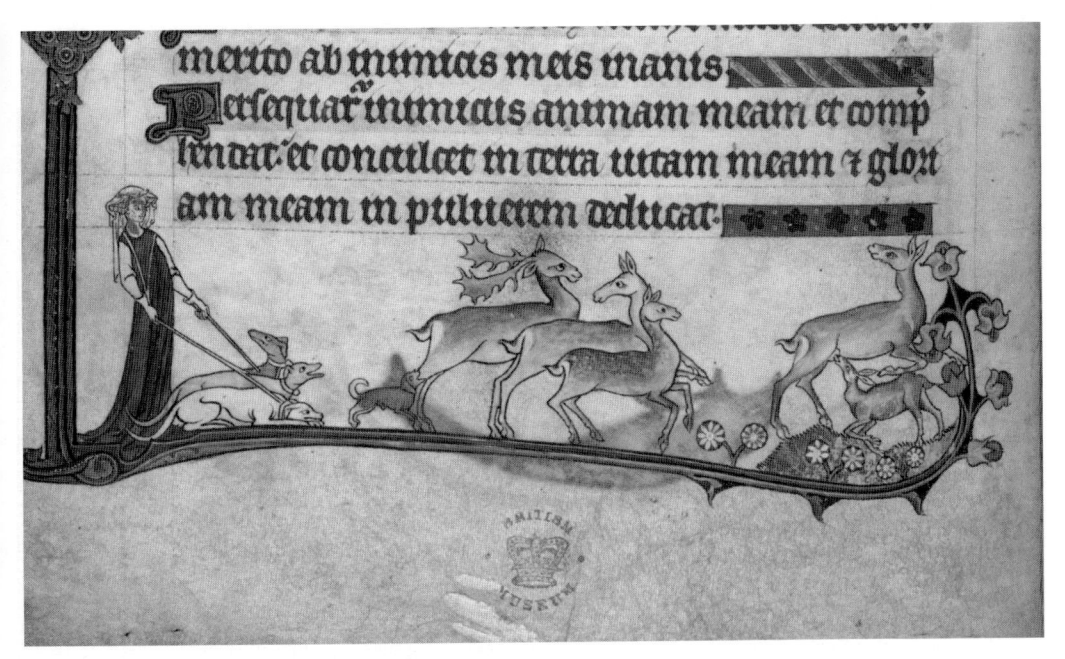

A noblewoman hunting, wearing a more elaborate veil and circlet, with her hair gathered at the sides; from the Alphonso Psalter, probably made to celebrate the proposed marriage of Edward I's son Alfonso of Bayonne (1273-84) in 1281. (BL Additional MS. 24686, fo. 13v; made available under a Public Domain Mark)

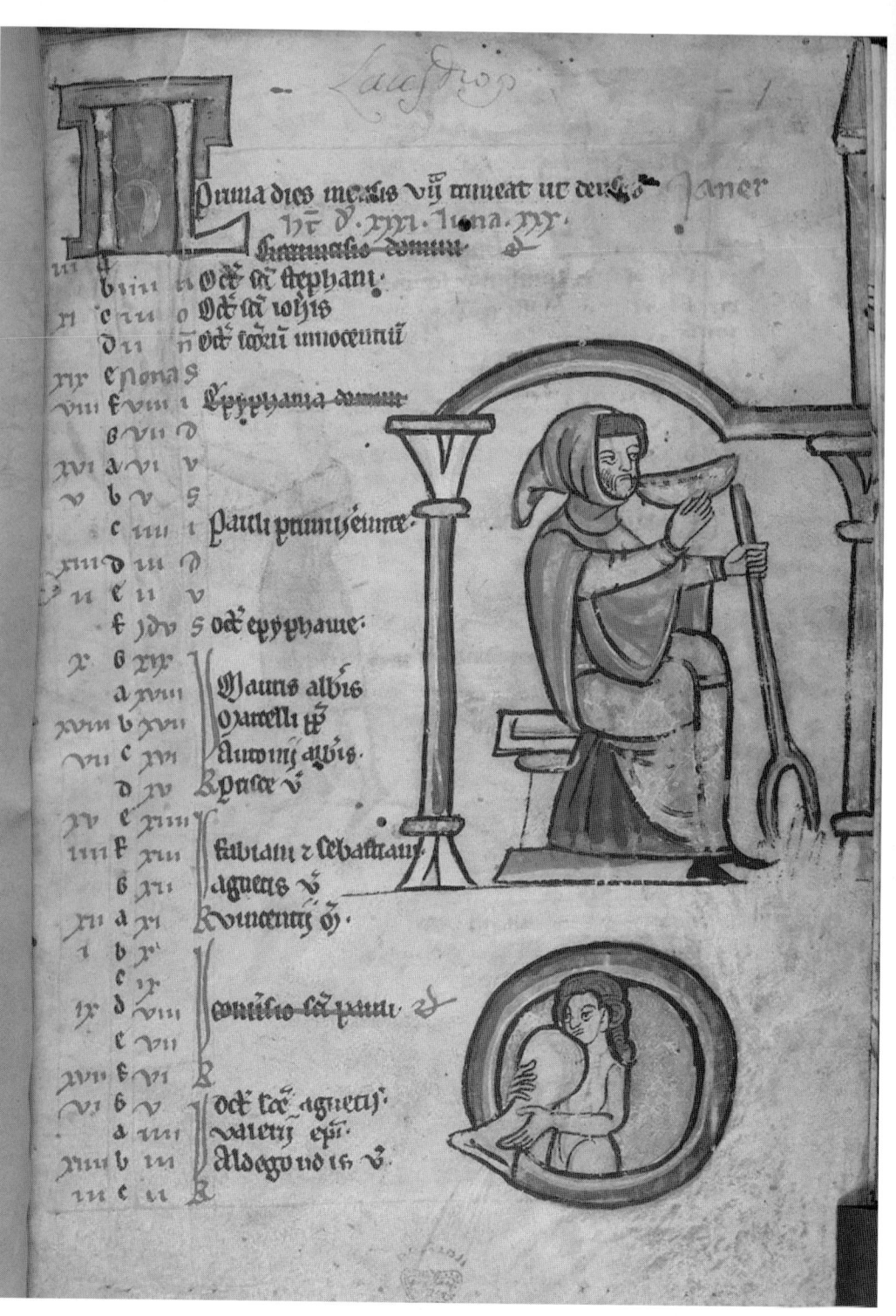

A man and a woman drinking, from a thirteenth-century psalter; the man wears a hooded cloak and the woman is naked. (BL Additional MS. 21114, fo. 1; made available under a Public Domain Mark)

Edvin Loach, Worcestershire in December 1393, three male attendees 'could hardly walk out of the church' after imbibing strong wine.[19]

Baptisms sometimes caused family disagreements. Lady Katherine Cobham was riding to the baptism of her nephew William Bonevyle in Shute, Devon on 31 August 1392, when she encountered Edward Dygher, a servant of her brother-in-law, who asked her where she was going. On hearing the reply, Edward told her, grinning, and with far more familiarity than one might expect from a servant to a knight's widow, '*Kate, Kate, ther to by myn pate, comyst ow to late*' ('thereto, by my pate [head], come you too late'). Katherine had assumed she would be asked to be her nephew's godmother, and was so angry that she rode home and refused to talk to her sister and brother-in-law for six months. And baptisms also caused some people to overspend. In London in 1382, it was proclaimed that 'whereas folks of the higher class in the said city, as well at the baptism of children as at the marriages of their children, have given large sums of money; through whose example, folks of lower rank have given just the same as people of higher rank, in impoverishment of the ordinary classes of the city aforesaid', no one in the city would be henceforth be allowed to give a gift worth more than 40d at any baptism.[20]

Purification

Approximately thirty or forty days after giving birth, women went through a ceremony called 'purification' or 'churching', which was the first time they went to church and participated in Mass again after the birth. The Purification of the Virgin Mary on 2 February, forty days after 25 December, was one of the most important feast days of the year in medieval England. Simon Pakeman's mother Alice gave birth to him in Kirby, Leicestershire on 20 March 1306 and was purified on 15 May, an unusually long time afterwards. Alice Selwyne was churched on 21 September 1403 after giving birth to her son William in Selmeston, Sussex on 24 August, and the following year also in Sussex, Margery Tauk was churched on 28 October after the birth of her son Robert on 23 September. Pernell, mother of Alice St Omer, was purified five weeks after giving birth on 25 March 1340. Katherine Montacute, née Grandisson, was purified on 14 August 1328 after giving birth to her son William Montacute (d. 1397), later Earl of Salisbury, on 19 June; also an unusually long time afterwards. William Herham's wife and his wife's daughter from her previous marriage (the women's names were not recorded) gave birth to children almost on the same day in Great Sanford, Essex in late 1308, and were purified together on 3 February 1309. William was twenty-nine at the time, and his wife, given that she had a daughter old enough to give birth herself, must have been rather older.[21]

Sir John Grey (d. 1359), nobleman and landowner, and a founder member of Edward III's Order of the Garter in 1349, was born in Rotherfield, Oxfordshire on 29 October 1300, and his parents John and Margaret held a great feast to celebrate Margaret's purification on 30 November. In the 1320s, locals still remembered this feast, and how almost all the abbots, priors and other 'good men' of the district attended it. Robert Welle was born in 'a great chamber by the hall towards the west' in Blatherwycke, Northamptonshire on the morning of 1 January 1297. His mother Joan invited all the residents of the village to dine with her when she was purified. After his younger daughter and co-heir Isabel was born on 31 May 1326, Sir John Moeles went hunting in Stoke Trister, Somerset, 'to take venison for a feast on the day of his wife's purification from the said Isabel his daughter', and after Maud Botiller gave birth to her son John in Pembridge, Herefordshire on 7 July 1387, Pembridge resident John Horsnet 'sold the father a red cow for the churching of Maud'. Roger Bailly sold Maud's husband a tun of Gascon wine for the ceremony. Sir Nicholas Kyriel sent a servant across the Channel to Ypres to buy robes for his wife Rose and himself to wear during her purification after giving birth to their son John in Walmer, Kent in October 1307.[22]

Wet-Nurses

Although working women tended to breastfeed their own children, the wives of barons, knights and landowners preferred to hire wet-nurses, and a woman of the locality who happened to be feeding her own infant was chosen. Juliana Catesby married her husband Hugh in Weldon Basset, Northamptonshire in the spring of 1333, and gave birth to their first son a year later on 25 April 1334. She was hired as the nurse of John Aylesbury, born in Weldon Basset on 6 May 1334. Millicent Ile bore her son, John, sometime in 1341 in Faldingworth, Lincolnshire, and at the end of September that year was hired as the wet-nurse of John Nevill. The unnamed Essex nurse who fed Agnes Den, born in early 1273,

Pregnancy and Childbirth (3)

also fed Ralph Jocelyn, born nearly two years later in December 1274. Edda Matlak of Ashleyhay in Derbyshire, who had borne an illegitimate daughter named Alice to William Hopton on 2 February 1286, was hired as the wet-nurse of John Derle a year later.[23]

When Lionel Coppeley was born in Leeds during the night of 21 April 1422, his father Richard sent a man to the house of Margaret Parcour to ask her to come and feed him. After the birth of Joan Wybbury in Cockington, Devon on 10 August 1424, her maternal grandmother Isabel Gorgeys summoned a man named John Estboughden to her, and said 'I am told that your wife is the best nurse in these parts, and so I ask that she be with me, at my hospitality, to nurse the daughter of my daughter. I will reward her for her labour and service, so that she is well content'. Isabel then gave John permission to attend her granddaughter's baptism, and afterwards, he told her that little Joan Wybbury was 'exceedingly beautiful' and that he would talk to his wife. Sixty-year-old John Lyndraper of Banbury in Oxfordshire stated in March 1356 that his sister Alice had been appointed as the wet-nurse of the infant Maud Stafford fifteen years earlier 'altogether against his will', though did not explain why he was so opposed to it. Alice nursed Maud for two years in the house of Thomas Deyestere, presumably her husband. After Henry Beaumont, son of John Beaumont and Katherine Everingham, was born in Folkingham Castle in Lincolnshire on 16 August 1381, John Ouseby, who lived a couple of miles away, 'had a discussion with the midwife and other women, through which they found a good wet-nurse' for the little boy.[24]

Not all women produced enough milk to feed their infants. Christina Archer gave birth to her son William Alkham in Kent on 8 September 1354, and asked Thomas Marrigge, one of her husband's officials, if he could provide a wet-nurse, as she 'had no milk to nourish her child'. If a mother produced insufficient milk and no other local woman was feeding her infant, cows' milk was used instead. After Robert Constable was born in Holme-on-Spalding-Moor, Yorkshire in March 1423, his mother Agnes accepted a gift of two milk-cows from villager Robert Ripley 'to provide milk for the heir during his youth'. John Hornecastell of Wigginton, Oxfordshire sold two cows to Alice Blount in November 1422 for milk for her son Humphrey, and Thomas Smyth sold a 'red cow' to the father of Ellen Walweyn in Herefordshire in January 1426 for the same purpose.[25]

At least some medieval parents expected that the wet-nurses they hired should remain celibate. John Holland, future Earl of Huntingdon and Duke of Exeter, was born on 29 March 1395 in Dartington, Devon, the chief manor of his parents, John Holland senior (half-brother of Richard II) and Elizabeth of Lancaster (sister of the future Henry IV). John the father hired a local woman named Isabel Hugh to act as his son's wet-nurse, and told her husband, John Hugh, not to have marital relations with his wife for the duration. John Hugh, who was about twenty-three at the time, took himself off to Guernsey in the Channel Islands and remained there for three years.[26] Laurence, the elder son of Robert and Alice Pavely, was born in Bingham, Nottinghamshire on 25 July 1327, and his godfathers were brothers named William and Thomas of Bingham. A few weeks after Laurence's birth, Thomas of Bingham was found in bed with Laurence's nurse, whose name is not recorded, and Thomas's kinsman John Poigne 'assisted in taking the said Thomas', i.e. removing him from the household and from the nurse's company.[27] Unfortunately no more information is available to tell us the fate of Thomas and his lover the unnamed nurse, though John Poigne was still alive in 1348, aged about sixty, when he related this story. Alice atte Market of Alford in Lincolnshire moved eighteen miles to Conisholme in April 1352 to work as the nurse of the newborn John Welle. While she was away, her husband William had an affair with an unnamed woman who worked as a maid in the village of Skendleby, five miles from Alford, which resulted in an illegitimate daughter. The nineteen-year-old son of the household where the woman worked agreed to become the little girl's godfather.[28]

Family Size

In an age centuries before reliable contraception, families were often quite large. Alice Ram of Kent was born on 21 October 1349, married Robert Freman at age eighteen, and gave birth to her eldest son, John Freman, around Christmas 1370 when she was twenty-one. She and Robert had eleven other sons and daughters.[29] William Hedrisham of London, who died in the plague year of 1349, stated in his will that he had seven brothers and two sisters. John Gisors, mayor of London three times in the 1310s, had four younger brothers and four sisters, and William Wyght, a fishmonger of London who died in 1395, had

Pregnancy and Childbirth (3)

four daughters and four sons. When George Knesworth, a draper, died in 1477, he left four sons and five daughters, all of them underage, though by 1495 three of the siblings were dead.[30] In 1357, William Langynow and Edith Squyers of Salisbury had been married for seven years and already had five children.[31]

Edward I's queen Leonor of Castile (b. c. November 1241) was the twelfth of her father Fernando III's fifteen children, seven sons and three daughters born to his first wife Beatriz and four sons and one daughter born to his second wife Jeanne. Leonor herself gave birth to at least four sons and ten daughters, perhaps five sons and eleven daughters. She married Edward in the autumn of 1254 and bore her youngest child, Edward II, in the spring of 1284 when she was forty-two. Edward I married his twenty-year-old second wife, Marguerite of France, in 1299 when he was sixty, and with her had another three children, the youngest born in May 1306 the month before Edward's sixty-seventh birthday. Edward I's eldest child was half a century older than his youngest. Edward and Leonor's grandson Edward III and his wife Philippa of Hainault had five daughters and seven sons, the eldest born in 1330 and the youngest in 1355, and the king had another three children with his mistress Alice Perrers in the 1360s.

There was an age gap of twenty-one years between brothers Robert and Simon Doulle of Buxlow, Suffolk, born in about 1253 and 1274, one of twenty-seven years between the siblings Thomas and Avelina Warde also of Buxlow, born in about 1247 and 1274, and one of twenty-nine years between the siblings William and Juliana Fraunk of Saxton in Yorkshire, born in about 1319 and 1348. William Eseby, born in Whorlton, Yorkshire in October 1331, had a much older brother, or perhaps half-brother, called John, who was already thirty-two when he was born, and William Stretton of Abbots Bromley in Staffordshire was twenty-three years older than his sister Katherine, born in October 1347. Thomas Ragged of Derbyshire died not long before 9 November 1293. His first wife was called Garciana and with her he had a daughter Maud, aged over thirty in 1293; he then married Margery and had three more daughters, Joan, aged fifteen in 1293, a daughter, whose name is missing, who was fourteen, and twelve-year-old Agnes; and his third wife, whose name is also missing, was pregnant when he died. When Robert Warde died in early 1307, he had a thirty-two-year-old married daughter, Joan Meynhill, from his first marriage and a nine-year-old daughter, Margaret

Warde, from his second, and his widow Ida was pregnant. The jurors who took part in Robert's inquisition post mortem stated, with a certain degree of obviousness, that they 'do not know whether it is of the male or female sex before it is born'.[32]

Parents' Ages

It is very difficult to ascertain people's ages, hundreds of years before birth certificates were invented and before parishes routinely began to record baptisms in the sixteenth century, though we do have some evidence. The children of people who held land directly from the king, and whose landowning parent died when the children were underage, had to prove their age when they were old enough to enter their late parent's lands. Men came of age at twenty-one, married women at fourteen, and unmarried women at sixteen. Many hundreds of these proofs of age still exist, and the jurors who took part in them and confirmed the heir's date of birth also had to provide their own ages. From this evidence, we can often determine how old people were, at least approximately, at key points in their lives such as when they married or became fathers, though as all the jurors were men it is, unfortunately, the case that we only rarely know women's ages.

Anselm Ide was in his late thirties when his wife Katherine bore their first son, William, in Kent in 1328, Adam Thorbrand was thirty-eight when his wife Amabel gave birth to their son William in Yorkshire in 1289, and John Honald was about forty-five when his son Robert was born in Acton Burnell, Shropshire in 1375. Sir John Pulteney (d. 1349), mayor of London three times in the 1330s, was old enough to act as an attorney in 1316 and must have been at least twenty-one then, so he was born in or before the mid-1290s. His son and heir William Pulteney was born sometime between October 1340 and March 1341. John atte Well was thirty-seven when he married Agnes atte Lynde in Ifield, Sussex on 18 September 1358, and Agnes's brother William atte Lynde was twenty-six when his son Robert was born on the same day.[33]

As noted in Chapter 2, there was little incentive for people to marry and quickly produce offspring unless the female partner was an heiress, such as Margaret Beaufort, who gave birth to her son Henry VII at the start of her teens. It may be significant that Margaret had no more children; perhaps this too-early consumption, pregnancy and childbirth damaged

Pregnancy and Childbirth (3)

her physically. Another example of early pregnancy and childbirth by an older husband is Isabella Verdon. She was born in Amesbury Priory, Wiltshire, on 21 March 1317, eight months after the death of her father Theobald, a wealthy landowner in the Midlands. Isabella and her older half-sisters Joan, Elizabeth and Margery Verdon were co-heirs to their father's sizable estate. Around 1328/30, Isabella was married to Henry, Lord Ferrers of Groby in Leicestershire, who was born c. 1303. Ferrers claimed his marital rights very early; as Isabella was an heiress, albeit one who had to share her inheritance with three others, Ferrers had an interest in producing a child with her as quickly as possible. No further details are known, but Isabella's mother Elizabeth sent her a gift for her purification in March 1331, the month of her fourteenth birthday, so Isabella must have given birth about forty days earlier. Unsurprisingly, the child born to a mother who was still only thirteen did not live, though Isabella gave birth to at least three younger children who survived into adulthood, including her and Henry's heir William Ferrers, born on 28 February 1333 three weeks before Isabella turned sixteen.[34]

Joan Montacute was the only surviving child and heir of Alice of Norfolk (c. 1324–51), herself one of the two co-heirs of her father the Earl of Norfolk. Joan was born on 2 February 1349, married William Ufford, later Earl of Suffolk, in or before 1359 when she was ten or younger, and was said to be pregnant on 14 February 1363, just days after her fourteenth birthday. Ufford, born in May 1338, was then almost twenty-five. This infant did not live, and Joan and Ufford had no other surviving children.[35] Other men, however, preferred to wait until their heiress wife was older. Isabel Chauncy, who inherited lands in Nottinghamshire and Lincolnshire, was born in March 1321 and lost her father Gerard when she was a year old. Sir Bertram Mountboucher purchased her marriage rights in July 1322, and Isabel married George Mountboucher, Bertram's nephew or younger son, at an unknown date. She gave birth to their son Nicholas Mountboucher in April 1342 at the age of twenty-one.[36]

Some boys were deemed physically and emotionally mature enough to consummate their marriages at fourteen, often when they were married to girls or young women older than they were. Richard II's widow Isabelle de Valois (b. 9 November 1389) married her cousin Charles of Angoulême (b. 24 November 1394), later Duke of Orléans, in June 1406 when they were sixteen and eleven. She gave birth to their daughter Jeanne on 13 September 1409, nine months and nineteen days after Charles's fourteenth birthday. Isabelle died shortly after the birth, so Charles not only became a father at age fourteen, but also a widower. Edmund Arundel, the only child of Richard, later Earl of Arundel, and his first wife Isabella Despenser, was apparently born in 1326: he was said to be eighteen in late 1344 and twenty in early 1347. According to their own testimony, Richard was seven and Isabella was eight when they wed in February 1321, and if their and their son's ages were correctly recorded, Richard was thirteen and Isabella was fourteen when they became parents.[37] Richard's son John Arundel from his second marriage was also a very young father.

When Henry, son and heir of Pernel and Conan Kelkefeld, was born in Yorkshire in September 1278, it was said that 'Conan the said heir's father was of such tender age when the said heir's mother was pregnant that it was commonly said he could not have begotten a child, and after the heir's birth there was much talk about it'.[38] Unfortunately, Conan's age was not recorded, but it sounds as though he was no more than twelve or thirteen and that his wife Pernel was some years older. Other young fathers were John Dinham of Devon, whose eldest child Joan was born in May or early June 1311 when he, born on 14 September 1295, was still fifteen, and John Jay of Shermanbury in Sussex, whose daughter Alice was born in November 1341 when John was also fifteen. William Plaunke, a landowner in Leicestershire, Wiltshire and Buckinghamshire, was born in late September 1325, and Katherine, the eldest of his three daughters, was born on 6 January 1341; she was conceived when William was fourteen.[39] In other cases, couples waited until the male partner was sixteen, and it is probably not a coincidence that Lionel of Antwerp and Elizabeth de Burgh's only child, Philippa, was born on 16 August 1355, thirty-seven weeks after Lionel's sixteenth birthday. Robert Colville was born in Bawdsey, Suffolk on 19 October 1304, nine months and a few weeks after his father Edmund's sixteenth birthday on 25 January 1304.[40]

Chapter 12

Illegitimacy

Illegitimacy was so extraordinarily common that numerous popes regularly handed out dispensations to forty or fifty aspiring clerics born out of wedlock at a time, and sometimes as many as a hundred.[1] The papal registers are full of dispensations granted to clerics and priests 'on account of illegitimacy' or because a cleric was 'the illegitimate son of a married man'. The word 'bastard' was often used as a second name by those born out of wedlock, or was imposed on them; among numerous other examples were Richard Bastard in the 1310s, who was an attorney, William Bastard of Devon in the 1330s, and John Bastard of London in the 1450s.[2]

Any child born to a married couple was deemed to be the husband's child unless proved otherwise, and there are therefore far fewer examples of a person being described as the 'illegitimate son of a married woman'.[3] This does not necessarily mean that it never or rarely happened, only that no one found out, and Pope Clement VI granted a series of dispensations in early 1335 to people whose mothers were married to men who were not their fathers. 'Peter, son of William Schaston of Kempston' in the diocese of Lincoln was called 'illegitimate son of a married woman', as were John Rotecod of Wimborne in the diocese of Salisbury, John Hakun of the diocese of Lincoln, and William Skydemar of the diocese of Llandaff in Wales. Thomas Chiteris, clerk of the diocese of Lincoln, was also called the 'illegitimate son of a married woman' in the 1340s. Thomas, Earl of Lancaster (d. 1322) had an illegitimate son, also called Thomas, with an unnamed woman 'of whom it is doubted whether at the time he was begotten she was married or a spinster'.[4] In 1444, lawyer John Heydon (d. 1479) of Norfolk disavowed his wife Eleanor's second son, and threatened to cut off her nose and kill the child if they came near him.[5]

Sex and Sexuality in Medieval England

It was extremely common for noblemen to father illegitimate children. John de Warenne, Earl of Surrey (1286–1347) had no children from his forty-year marriage to Edward I's French granddaughter Jeanne de Bar (c. 1295–1361) and was the last Warenne Earl of Surrey, though did father at least nine illegitimate children, six sons and three daughters (and had an illegitimate half-brother who joined the Church and whose name was also John). The earl's two known mistresses, Maud Nerford and Isabelle Holland, were of high birth: Maud was the niece of Lord Ros of Helmsley, and Isabelle's brother Sir Thomas Holland married Edward I's granddaughter Joan of Kent and was the father of Richard II's half-siblings. We are lucky that Warenne made strenuous (though unsuccessful) efforts in 1316 and again in 1344 to annul his marriage to Jeanne de Bar and wed one of his lovers instead, and that he ignored Jeanne in his will and referred to Isabelle Holland as his *compaigne* or wife, as otherwise, we might not know the women's identities.[6]

Ralph Stafford (1301–72), the first Earl of Stafford in 1351, had an illegitimate son named Thomas, who joined the Church. Thomas's legitimate half-brother Hugh, later the second Earl of Stafford, petitioned the pope on his behalf in 1364.[7] Thomas Beauchamp, Earl of Warwick (1314–69), as well as fathering sixteen children with his wife Katherine Mortimer (d. 1369), had an illegitimate son called John Athereston, and Sir Walter Manny (*c.* 1310–72), second husband of Margaret, Countess of Norfolk and father of Anne, Countess of Pembroke, had two illegitimate daughters who bore the unusual and poetic names of Mailosel and Malplesant.[8] Laurence Hastings, Earl of Pembroke (1320–48), had a half-brother named Sir William Hastings (d. 1349), illegitimate son of his father John (1286–1325), and was extremely close to him.[9] William used his father's name, and some other illegitimate people did the same, though it was more common for people born outside marriage to use their mothers' names, as John Athereston presumably did. People who appeared on record as the child of a woman, such as 'Walter, son of Beatrice Gomme', a criminal from Guildford in Surrey, and 'Thomas, son of Sarah Bredmongestere', arrested for disturbing the peace in London, were invariably illegitimate.[10] The Norfolk knight Sir John Reppes (d. 1373) had illegitimate sons called John Martyn and Gregory Scarlet, presumably their mothers' names, and the illegitimate son of Richard Blount of Bedfordshire (d. 1390) was called William Whyte. King Henry IV fathered an illegitimate son in 1401 named Edmund Lebourde.[11] William Newenham of London, who died in the plague year of 1349, had an illegitimate daughter named Agnes Dolfyn whose mother was also named Agnes Dolfyn, and had two more illegitimate children, John and Joan Blaket, with Maud Blaket.[12]

One of the very few medieval English noblewomen we know who gave birth to an illegitimate child was Constance of York (*c.* 1374/75–1416), a granddaughter of two kings. Constance's father was Edmund of Langley (1341–1402), first Duke of York, the fifth son of Edward III; her mother was Isabel of Castile (1355-92), youngest daughter of King Pedro I 'the Cruel' of Castile and Leon.[13] Constance's husband Thomas Despenser, Lord of Glamorgan and briefly Earl of Gloucester from 1397 to 1399, was executed in January 1400, and the widowed Constance had an affair some years later with the young Earl of Kent, Edmund Holland, born in 1383 and a few years her junior. This relationship resulted in the birth of an illegitimate daughter, Alianore Holland, in *c.* 1405, who married James Tuchet, Lord Audley (b. 1397).

We would not know the true circumstances of Alianore's birth except that in 1431 she launched an audacious claim to be the heir of her late father (d. 1408), stating that she was his legitimate child. The Earl of Kent's heirs were in fact his two surviving sisters, the dowager Duchesses of York and Clarence, and the children and grandchildren of his other three sisters. They all worked together to deny Alianore's claim, pointing out that her mother Constance attended Kent's wedding to Lucia Visconti of Milan in 1407, but did not speak out and declare that Kent was already married to her. They called their kinswoman 'Alianore, wyf to James lord Audeley, pretendyng, namyng and affermyng herself doghter and heir to þe said Edmond late erle of Kent, and begetyn and born in espousels pretentyd had betwix hym and Custance, of late wyf to Thomas lord Spencer'.[14] Why Alianore's parents did not marry on learning of Constance's pregnancy, given that Edmund Holland, as an earl and a half-nephew of the late Richard II, was of high enough rank to marry Constance, is rather hard to explain. It may be that Henry IV forbade the match because Edmund was loyal to him, whereas Constance openly opposed Henry.

The extra-marital relationship between Constance of York and Edmund Holland is a rather interesting one for another reason: Constance's mother Isabel of Castile might have had an affair in the

1380s with Edmund's uncle John Holland, half-brother of Richard II. This is not certain, but there was a close connection between the two: in her will, Isabel left Holland a number of bequests, and bequeathed to her son Edward some valuable items which Holland had given her. The manuscript copyist John Shirley, who worked for many years for Isabel of Castile's grandson-in-law the Earl of Warwick, wrote that John Holland loved Isabel.[15] In 1386, Holland married Isabel's niece-in-law Elizabeth of Lancaster, probably after making her pregnant while she was married to the barely adolescent Earl of Pembroke. Holland's busy sex life continued: he fathered an illegitimate son named William Huntingdon, whose name must mean that he was born after Holland received the earldom of Huntingdon in June 1388, during his marriage to Elizabeth.[16]

Lucy Thweng was born in 1279, and inherited lands in Yorkshire from her father Robert.[17] Lucy's life was almost impossibly dramatic: she was married three times, abducted twice, and, while attempting to have her first marriage to William Latimer annulled, was accused before an ecclesiastical court of committing adultery with Nicholas Meinill or Meynille.[18] Supposedly, Lucy gave birth to a son in December 1294 barely four months after her wedding to William Latimer, and doubts were cast on the boy's legitimacy, though an inquisition taken in March 1327 states that Lucy and Latimer's son was then only twenty-five or twenty-six.[19] Lucy was abducted from William Latimer in 1303, though perhaps she left her husband willingly, and she subsequently had a relationship with Sir Nicholas Meinill which resulted in a son also named Nicholas. She gained an annulment of her marriage to William Latimer, separated from Nicholas Meinill in 1310 and married Sir Robert Everingham, but Meinill was unhappy about this and abducted her in or before January 1313. Everingham died in 1316, and by 1318 Lucy was married to her third husband, Bartholomew Fanacourt. Despite her son Nicholas's illegitimacy, Nicholas Meinill the elder, who had no legitimate children, made him heir to his lands.[20] To complete this fascinating family history, Nicholas Meinill (the elder)'s mother Christina was accused in 1290 of committing adultery with Walter Hamerton and 'W. Grenefeud' or Greenfield.[21]

At the lower levels of society, it was far easier for women to have extra-marital relationships and illegitimate children. In the mid-1280s in Ashleyhay, Derbyshire, Edda Matlak and William Hopton had a relationship which resulted in an illegitimate daughter named Alice, born on 2 February 1286.[22] Isabel Moleseye and John Gildesburgh of London (d. 1349) had three illegitimate daughters, Margaret, Isabel and Juliana, and John himself was illegitimate.[23] Alice Moton (d. 1360), daughter and heir of Robert Moton of London, had an illegitimate daughter named Emma with John Vykery, and although the couple married two years after Emma's birth, Emma was still deemed illegitimate and thus ineligible to inherit her mother's properties.[24] Another London resident, Katherine St Albans, had a long-term relationship with Master Richard Gloucester, parson of Stevenage in Hertfordshire and a lawyer, in the 1310s and 1320s. Despite being a clergyman, Richard fathered two sons during his long relationship with Katherine: John, born in 1317, and Nicholas, born in 1319. In his will of November 1328, Master Richard left his house in Friday Street, London to Katherine for the rest of her life, and appointed her as the guardian of their children, whom he named as his will only as her sons, not his own. John and Nicholas were, however, acknowledged as Richard's sons by the London authorities, and they both used his name and inherited his property. Katherine St Albans lived openly with Master Richard Gloucester for many years, and the fact that they had children together was widely known, yet there is no evidence anywhere of any censure or punishment. Katherine's father was named Geoffrey, though she sometimes appeared on record as 'the daughter of Isabel St Albans', so was herself probably also born out of wedlock.[25]

Henry I (r. 1100–35), William the Conqueror's youngest son, holds the record among medieval English kings for fathering the most illegitimate children, and his great-grandson King John (r. 1199–1216) had at least a dozen. A few of Henry I's many illegitimate children made brilliant marriages; his daughter Sybilla, for instance, married King Alexander I of Scotland, and Maud (not to be confused with her legitimate half-sister of the same name, Holy Roman Empress and mother of Henry II) married the Duke of Brittany. Later in the Middle Ages, however, attitudes changed, and children born outside marriage married well down the social scale. Joan, only legitimate child and heir of Piers Gaveston, Earl of Cornwall (d. 1312) died unmarried in early 1325 around the time of her thirteenth birthday, but had been betrothed firstly to Thomas Wake, an influential nobleman who was the great-great-grandson of an emperor of Constantinople, and secondly to

John Multon, a grandson of the Earl of Ulster and heir to his father's extensive lands in northern England. By contrast, Joan's half-sister Amie, Gaveston's illegitimate daughter, married John Driby, an archer. Maud, elder daughter and co-heir of Henry of Grosmont, first Duke of Lancaster, married her second husband Wilhelm von Wittelsbach, Duke of Bavaria and a son of the Holy Roman Emperor, in 1352. Maud's younger sister Blanche married Edward III's son John of Gaunt and was the mother of Henry IV. Their half-sister Juliane (d. after 1407), Duke Henry's illegitimate daughter, married William Danet, a tax collector of Leicester.

As well as marrying down, illegitimate children in England had no claim to their parents' inheritance if it was held in chief, i.e. directly from the king. When Edmund Vauncy, a landowner in Cambridgeshire, died in August 1372, his heir was named in his inquisition post mortem as his son Edmund the younger, born c. November 1367. This younger Edmund himself died in March 1390, leaving his widow Clarice 'secretly pregnant' (why her pregnancy was 'secret' was not explained). Edmund's twenty-seven-year-old sister Joan and her husband Thomas Priour, however, claimed that Edmund had been illegitimate, and had 'intruded himself' into lands that rightfully belonged to Joan as her father's only legitimate child. In the 1390s, Richard 'Basset' claimed to be the heir of Sir Ralph Basset, but turned out to be the illegitimate son of a monk of Croxden Abbey named Thomas Leke and his lover Isabel Lowekyn.[26] John Iselbek died in c. 1317, and his son William, whose mother was 'one Amabel, a Scot' and was himself born in Scotland, entered into his lands in the north of England. Years later, it transpired that William was illegitimate and had no right to the inheritance. The matter was still under discussion as late as 1344.[27]

When John Wygeton of Cumberland died in 1315, his heir was his twenty-two-year-old daughter Margaret Crekedek. John's five sisters and their children, however, claimed that Margaret's mother Denise had been precontracted to a man named John Paynel before she married John Wygeton and that Margaret was therefore illegitimate. The matter was finally resolved in 1321 when the Bishop of London (London being Margaret's birthplace) declared that Margaret was John Wygeton's 'lawful daughter ... and not a bastard'. An inquisition was held in 1319 to determine whether John Gadesden and Christina Stane's daughter Edith was legitimate, and whether she had a claim to her mother's estate

Illegitimacy

in Wiltshire, Hampshire and Bedfordshire. It turned out that Christina and John had an affair after Christina's husband Peter Stane died, and as they never married, Edith was not one of her mother's co-heirs. Christina's estate passed to her three legitimate daughters by Peter, Edith's half-sisters. The elderly Thomas Trot, landowner in Norfolk, Kent, Middlesex, Surrey and Sussex, died in September 1355. Before dying, Thomas stated that he had never had legitimate children, that his only wife Agnes was 'of great age' when they married, and that his heir was his late brother's daughter Christina. An inquisition in 1383 found, however, that Thomas had married Alice Luggere in Mayfield, Sussex, and with her had a son named John Trot, born in the 1330s, his rightful heir.[28] Perhaps Thomas suffered from dementia and had forgotten his first wife and their son, or remembered his son but forgot that he had been married before and that John was legitimate.

Many people did their best to provide well for their lovers and their illegitimate children after their deaths. John Ashford, a woolmonger of London who died in 1329, fathered six illegitimate children, two sons and four daughters, with two women. With Joan Stodleye, John had Thomas Mordale, Alice and Joan; and with Lettice Bilham, he had John, Katherine and Isabel. Ashford left generous bequests of money and property to all his children and both of his lovers in his will. His daughter Joan married the haberdasher John Levynge in 1335 and received £20 left to her by her father as her generous dowry, and Joan's full brother Thomas Mordale was a mercer who was still alive in 1363. Their half-brother John, who unlike Thomas used their father's name, died in 1356, leaving Thomas his shops in London and £15 in cash. Relations between John Ashford's two out-of-wedlock families appear to have been perfectly amicable. Thomas Albon, also a woolmonger of London, left certain unspecified bequests to his illegitimate children John and Elizabeth as well as to his legitimate children John and Alice on his death in 1392. When the illegitimate John died soon after his father, his portion of his father's goods passed instead to his sister Elizabeth.[29]

Henry Causton (d. 1350), a mercer, left bequests to his illegitimate daughter Katherine and her mother Isabella, gave Katherine 100 marks (£66.66) as her future dowry, and suggested that his wife Margaret might look after Katherine until she came of age, even though the girl's mother was alive. This was perhaps because Margaret Causton, who received

101

£300 in cash from her husband as well as all his movable goods and vessels, was far more well-off than Isabella, her husband's former lover. John Hardewyk died in the early 1400s, leaving a legitimate daughter named Alice and an illegitimate daughter named Isabella. Both girls were given into the custody of John's widow Katherine and her second husband John Frensshe in March 1405. William Shelton, a squire of Suffolk, died in 1421, and his heir was his seventeen-year-old son John, born to William's wife Katherine Baret. William also had, however, an illegitimate daughter named Amice, and ordered his executors and descendants to pay her 40s a year for the rest of her life.[30]

Chapter 13

Prostitution

As noted above, women who wished to live alone found it difficult to earn their own living, and often had to resort to selling sex. Medieval prostitution was, as one might expect, a choice women generally made 'under severe constraints'.[1] Although medieval theory held that women were naturally more lustful than men, rather contradictorily, men being allowed to have access to women who sold sex was considered a necessary safety valve for male sexuality, and it was deemed better in such cases for a man to sate his lusts with a woman already considered corrupt than to risk degrading his wife or committing adultery or rape. Even so, the number of prostitutes was tiny: Ruth Mazo Karras has calculated the number of women accused of prostitution in ecclesiastical courts in late fifteenth-century London as around fifty per year, or about 0.1 or 0.2% of the population of the diocese.[2]

There is considerable evidence for the practice of prostitution in London in the Middle Ages. At the beginning of the 1260s, there was a brothel in the parish of All Hallows Colemanescherche in London, where Margery Pyriton, Agnes Blida, Dulcia Trye, Maud of Norfolk, Notekina Hoggenhore and Isabel la Rus worked; they rented a house from Alice Blunde. Around the same time, another brothel was situated in Bishopsgate ward and Beatrice Wynton, Isabel Staunford and Margery Karl worked there, and in 1266/67 Dulcia Gravesend worked as a prostitute in London.[3] Prostitutes were officially forbidden to reside within the city walls of London in 1277/78, though some of them continued to do so. One of them, at the end of the 1290s, was Christine Gravesende. When she and 'other common prostitutes living in the city' were summoned to appear before the mayor and aldermen, she and 'a certain Robert Bonevil, her paramour' punched the mayor's serjeant Richard Peleter in the mouth. In 1281, four men – Roger Grascherche, Fulk Barbur, Hugh Barber and Walter Taillur – kept 'houses of ill fame' in London.[4]

Margaret Hontyngdone, resident of Broad Street ward in London, was imprisoned in a jail called the Tun on Cornhill in June 1311, on the grounds that she 'had been before driven out from the ward aforesaid as a common strumpet, and had afterwards harboured men of bad repute'. The following January, Margaret was imprisoned in the Tun again for 'being of bad character', and on this occasion was joined by Marion Honytone and Henry Beste, a man 'of bad repute'.[5] In the 1320s, Alice Wytteney was a 'courtesan' who rented a house from John Assheby in Billingsgate ward, and Emma Brakkele, said to be a 'harlot', worked in Fetter Lane a few years later. In February 1339, Geoffrey Perler went there to 'lie with her'.[6] William Cok, butcher of Cock Lane, was said to 'harbour prostitutes' in his houses (plural) in December 1300. Thomas, vicar of St Sepulchre without Newgate, and John Copersmyth, took matters into their own hands by breaking into the houses and tearing away eleven doors and five windows with hammers and chisels, and distributed them among William Cok's neighbours. William accused the men of trespass and criminal damage in the mayor's court, but was informed that Thomas and John's action was lawful. The same thing happened to Richard atte Nax in 1305: prostitutes dwelt in his house, so the prior of Holy Trinity and seven servants removed his doors and windows.[7] The beadle of Farringdon Without ward was accused in 1344 of accepting bribes 'from disorderly women to protect them in their practices', and an inquisition heard that Agnes Chedyngfeld and Clarice Claterballok 'are women of ill-fame, and that a certain Sayer Valoyns, who dwells with the latter, prefers bad company to good'. Clarice's last name presumably means that she specialised in clattering her clients' *balloks*. In November 1364, Joan, wife of William atte Grene, swore not to keep her house as a brothel.[8]

William Dalton was imprisoned for over two months in 1338 for 'keeping a house of ill-fame to which married women and their paramours and other bad characters resorted'. Robert Stratford was accused in July 1338 of keeping a brothel where women named as Alice Donbely and Alice Tredewedowe, and unnamed others, worked, and at the same time, Ellen Evesham of Fleet Street 'keeps a disorderly house and harbours thieves and prostitutes'. Sisters named Agnes and Juliane worked as prostitutes in Holborn, outside the city walls, in the late 1330s, and in 1344 'women of ill-fame' worked in houses belonging to Sir Richard Wylughby and William Sendale in Seacoal Lane. In July 1340, more 'women of ill-fame' were said to frequent a house belonging to James Sherman called *Breggehous* ('Bridge House'); John Catton 'keeps a common bawdy-house'; and Sarra Mareschal used the home she rented from the archdeacon of Colchester as a 'disorderly house'.[9]

The oddly-named Zenobius Martyn was indicted in January 1373 as a 'common bawd and associate of prostitutes'. He admitted that he welcomed into his house 'men of ill-fame, evildoers, thieves and prostitutes'.[10] The Middle English word *baud(e)* or 'bawd' meant a procurer or a pander, or in modern idiom, a pimp. Elizabeth Moring was punished by an hour locked in the public pillory followed by permanent exile from London in 1386 after being convicted of being a 'common harlot and procuress' and of selling the sexual services of her female servants. Publicly, Elizabeth pretended to hire apprentices in the craft of embroidery, but instead forced the women to 'live a lewd life'.[11] This was, sadly, far from the only case of forced prostitution in medieval London. In 1439, Margaret Hathewyk and Margery Bradley took Isabella Lane and another unnamed girl to the house of merchants from Lombardy, who had paid the two women to 'deflower the said [Isabella] against her will'. The poor girl was then taken to the stews in Southwark (see paragraph below) for three days 'to be used in lustful acts'.[12] Another appalling crime does at least reveal the existence of male prostitutes in medieval London. Sometime between 1276 and 1321, a chaplain purchased the sexual favours of a young man, and they went to the church of All Saints Barking. After they were finished, the chaplain sodomised the unfortunate young man with a stick, and inflicted a mortal injury.[13]

Throughout the Middle Ages, the London authorities attempted to banish prostitutes from the city and to force them to work in the 'stews' or brothels of Southwark on the south bank of the Thames, which was called *Stewysside* or 'stew side'.[14] In December 1310, Edward II ordered the mayor, Richer Refham, and the sheriffs, Simon Corp and Peter Blakeney, to take measures for 'the suppression of houses of ill-fame' in London.[15] Whatever measures the men took were ineffectual. In the seventh year of Richard II's reign, June 1383 to June 1384, the London authorities issued regulations for the 'punishment of whoremongers, bawds, unchaste priests and adulterers'.[16] Male whoremongers (*putours* in the French original) and bawds would have their heads and beards shaved off except for 'a fringe on the head, two inches in breadth', and would be taken to the pillory accompanied by minstrels playing the trumpet or drums to draw everyone's attention to the victim. A second offence would result in the same punishment with ten days' imprisonment on top, and a third offence would be penalised by several hours on the pillory, ten days' imprisonment, and perpetual exile from London. Female bawds and keepers of brothels would be taken to the pillory, and her hair would be 'cut round about her head'. Subsequent offences were subject to the same punishment as male bawds. Courtesans, adulteresses and 'common scolds' were to be temporarily imprisoned, then taken to Aldgate (one of the great gates into London) wearing a striped hood and carrying a white wand. Minstrels would then accompany them to the pillory, and after an hour or two locked there, the minstrels would again accompany them through Cheapside and Newgate to Cock Lane, where they would take up abode. A second offence resulted in a woman's hair being cut off and another hour or two on the pillory, and a third in being cast out of London.

In 1393, Richard II and the mayor and aldermen of London made another attempt to force prostitutes out of the city. They stated that:

> ...many and diverse affrays, broils, and dissensions, have arisen in times past, and many men have been slain and murdered, by reason of the frequent resort of, and consorting with, common harlots, at taverns, brewhouses, and other places of ill-fame, within the said city, and the suburbs thereof; and more especially through Flemish women, who profess and follow such shameful and dolorous life.

Prostitutes were ordered to 'keep themselves to the places thereunto assigned, that is to say, the stews [*lestupbes*] on the other side of Thames, and Cock Lane, on pain of losing and forfeiting the upper garment that she shall be wearing, together with her hood, every time that any one of them shall be found doing to the contrary of this proclamation'. City officials were given permission to take 'such garments and hoods' and to bring them to the Guildhall. It was proclaimed in 1391 that 'no boatman bring man or woman to the stews between sunset and sunrise, nor moor his boat within 20 fathoms of the shore during that period, lest misdoers be assisted in their coming and going'.[17] Sometime in the fifth year of Henry V's reign, i.e. between 21 March 1417 and 20 March 1418, it was proclaimed in London that landlords and landladies must not rent out any property to 'any man or woman ... known to be of evil and vicious life'. This was done on the grounds that when such men and women were indicted and removed from the wards where they lived, they simply went to a neighbouring ward or to a city suburb in order to 'carry on the illicit works of their carnal appetites'. Furthermore, the proclamation thundered, they encouraged others to commit 'the most abominable deeds that one may think of or devise, to the very great and abominating displeasure of God'.[18]

Noble and royal households of the Middle Ages consisted almost entirely of men (the only exceptions were the lady's personal attendants, the nurses of any small children, and washerwomen), and servants in the royal household were not allowed to have their families living with them at court. In an ordinance made for the royal household in 1318, prostitutes were to be removed from the court, and were imprisoned for forty days if found there a third time.[19] This, given that the household consisted of a few hundred men who were not allowed to have their wives living with them, was clearly an ongoing issue.

Chapter 14

Ravishment and Abduction

Age of Consent

According to medieval canon law, girls could marry and consummate their marriage at age twelve and boys at age fourteen. The First Statute of Westminster in 1275 is considered to have set the age of consent in English law at twelve, where it would remain for exactly 600 years; it was raised to thirteen in 1875 and then to sixteen in 1885, where it has remained ever since (the age of consent for same-sex sex was set at twenty-one in 1967 and at sixteen in 2000). An age is not specifically given in the 1275 statute, but it states that the king forbade anyone to 'ravish or take by force a maiden within age', either with her consent or without.[1] 'Within age' is generally assumed to have been under twelve years old. This does not, however, mean that everyone, or even many people, did marry and have sex at the age of twelve, just as in modern Britain few people get married when they turn sixteen just because they are now legally able to do so. Regardless of what canon and civil law might have said, few medieval people considered a girl of twelve or thirteen to be a viable sexual partner (though there were some exceptions, as noted above).

It was far more usual for regular marital relations to be delayed until a girl was physically and emotionally mature enough to cope with intercourse, pregnancy and childbirth, and indeed to be physically mature enough to become pregnant in the first place. Edward II and Isabella of France married in January 1308 when Isabella was twelve, and conceived their first child, Edward III, a little over four years later; he was born in November 1312 when Isabella was seventeen or almost. Edward II, in common with most other medieval men, was unwilling to have sex with a barely pubescent girl. John Carmi Parsons has shown that the norm among the Plantagenet dynasty was to consummate a marriage at twelve, to make it legal and binding, but to delay regular conjugal relations until the girl was fifteen.[2] Henry III was born on 1 October 1207 and his queen Eleanor of Provence probably on 30 November 1222. When they wed in January 1236, Henry was twenty-eight and Eleanor only thirteen, and their eldest child Edward I was conceived in c. September 1238.[3] Henry VI (b. December 1421) received permission from Pope Eugene IV to consummate his marriage to Marguerite of Anjou (b. March 1430) 'on days when it is forbidden to so', on the grounds that Henry wished a 'speedy consummation' to ensure 'the peace and tranquillity of the realms of France and England'. Fifteen-year-old Marguerite arrived in England in April 1445, though Eugene's letter was sent in January, and mentioned that 'the sea voyage to England is during the winter apt to be prolonged by reasons of storms and tempests', causing delays to the couple's wedding and marital relations.[4] Henry's speedy consummation of his marriage did not, however, result in pregnancy, as he surely wished: the couple's only child, Edward of Lancaster, was not born until October 1453.

The wording of the First Statute of Westminster of 1275, that nobody must 'ravish or take by force a maiden within age', either with her consent or without, does make clear that later medieval England was well aware of the need for consent.[5] In September 1328, someone acting on Edward III's behalf – Edward was then only fifteen years old – sent three men to search for Joan Breton, and to determine 'whether it was against her will that she was ravished, abducted or detained' in Clipstone, Nottinghamshire. If they found that what had happened to Joan was without her consent, the three were 'to cause her to be safely and decently kept'.[6]

In or soon before July 1318, men in the retinue of the nobleman Hugh Despenser the Elder (1261–1326), later Earl of Winchester, broke into the home of George Percy, his son John, and his daughter-in-law Elizabeth née Hertrigg in the Wiltshire village of Great Chalfield. This raid was part of an ongoing feud between Despenser and the Percys, and in 1312 Despenser had abducted Elizabeth from the custody of George Percy, then her guardian and later her father-in-law. One of Despenser's knights who helped to carry out the 1318 raid was Sir Ingelram Berenger (*c.* 1265–1336). Berenger's son John accompanied him, and was accused of abducting and raping Elizabeth Percy, née Hertrigg. What is notable is the youth of both Elizabeth and John Berenger: Elizabeth was born in either 1303 or 1304 and was fourteen or fifteen at the time, and John was born c. 1304 and was also about fourteen. He 'surrendered himself to the king's peace and prison to stand to right' for his crime a year later, and owing to his youth was assigned a 'keeper for [his] safe-keeping'.[7]

Ravishment/Rape

The Latin word *rapuerunt* was used when Edward II ordered an inquest into Elizabeth Percy's ordeal. The word also sometimes appeared as *rapuit* or *raptus*, and another word used in medieval documents in England, this time in French, is *ravir*. These words can mean to ravish or to rape, but can also mean to seize, abduct, or take by force. In the summer of 1327, the former king Edward II, forced to abdicate his throne to his teenage son Edward III earlier that year, was held in captivity at Berkeley Castle in Gloucestershire, and a group of his followers attacked the castle and temporarily freed him. His guardian Lord Berkeley stated that the men had *ravi le pere nostre seignor le roi hors de nostre garde*, 'seized the father of our lord the king from our custody'.[8] In this context, *ravi* clearly does not mean raped. In many other contexts, however, the word did mean rape, and the modern English word 'rape' derives ultimately from Latin *rapere*, 'to seize'.[9] The frequent use of the word 'ravishment' in medieval England can be puzzling to us as it encompasses concepts we think of as separate: forced intercourse, abduction, and elopement, i.e. an 'abduction' that the woman in question consented to but that her parents or guardians did not.[10]

In the First Statute of Westminster, the punishment for rape was set at a mere two years' imprisonment and a fine, and the statute referred to 'ravishment or taking by force'. This was, however, a deliberately low sentence because the law on rape was undergoing a major change, and the Second Statute ten years later imposed the death penalty as the maximum sentence.[11] For the first time in English history, women were allowed to prosecute their attackers. In 1322, for example, Joan Eston prosecuted a clerk named Master Richard Bachiler of Warwickshire for rape before the King's Bench.[12] Susan Brownmiller's classic *Against Our Will* points out the giant leap forward in thinking taken by the Statutes of Westminster; our understanding of the concept of statutory rape, the rape of an underage girl where her alleged consent is immaterial, dates from these statutes. They also criminalised the rape of married, i.e. non-virgin,

Ravishment and Abduction

women, though the criminalisation of rape within marriage would have to wait for another 700 years. In his *On the Laws and Customs of England*, Bracton mentioned almost in passing the rape of 'matrons, nuns, widows, concubines and even prostitutes'. While modern readers might gnash their teeth at the 'even', it was a novel idea that women who were not virgins from noble landowning families could also be raped, and that this was a punishable felony.[13]

As noted above, however, if a rape victim was unfortunate enough to become pregnant as a result of her ordeal, it was held that she must have climaxed, and therefore had enjoyed the experience and had not been raped. And whether many women saw justice done, even if they were deemed not to have been raped because they had become pregnant, is another matter. Sometime before January 1350, though the location and circumstances are unclear, the unfortunate Elianore Merton was raped by three men, Nicholas Bolton, John Lavenham, and John Waltham. The rapists sent three separate petitions to Edward III, all written by different scribes, but with such similar wording that it is apparent that the three worked together to devise them. They all asked to be pardoned for their crime, which was called *ravissement* in the medieval French in which the petitions were written, on the grounds that they had done excellent service for the king during his military campaign in France in 1346/47. They all cited the Magna Carta, and two of them, Lavenham and Bolton, also declared, for some unclear reason, that the king should have regard for the soul of his late father Edward II and issue them a pardon. Their efforts paid off: in January 1350, Edward III duly pardoned the three and released them from prison 'in consideration of [their] good service' during his siege of Calais in 1347.[14]

Men could be, and often were, pardoned for serious crimes such as rape and homicide if they performed excellent military service for the king, and the case of the unfortunate Elianore Merton is just one example. Another is Katherine Byrom or Boyrom or Beyrom, 'ravished' by Alexander Wirkeslegh, Richard Lynhales, and John and Robert Holt in Staffordshire in 1350. Edward III pardoned the men because of their 'good service done in a late conflict on the sea against the Spaniards in the company of Edward, prince of Wales', a reference to the naval battle of Winchelsea on 29 August 1350. Richard Lynhales was pardoned for raping Katherine as early as 8 September 1350, just ten days after the battle, and his mother Maud was also pardoned for 'abetting and aiding' her son despite knowing that he had been indicted for rape. Alexander Wirkeslegh, evidently a most unpleasant piece of work, was pardoned for raping Katherine Byrom and another woman named Margery Jurdenson; for assaulting Henry Adorton and his servants; breaking into and stealing from several people's homes; killing horses and other animals belonging to John Trafford; 'and all manner of other homicides, felonies and trespasses done by him'. Finally, the brothers John and Robert Holt were pardoned for the murder of three men, and for raping Katherine and 'breaking the gates and doors of her father', implying that the men attacked her in her own family home.[15] Edward III required lots of men to fight in his endless wars against France and Scotland, and did not necessarily care too much what crimes his soldiers had committed; indeed, a lack of moral compass was perhaps deemed a bonus. His grandsons Richard II and Henry IV, on the other hand, often pardoned men for all felonies they had committed except murder, rape, and treason.[16]

At a parliament held in Westminster in October 1382, Sir Thomas and Alice West presented a petition to John of Gaunt, Duke of Lancaster, uncle of fifteen-year-old Richard II and the most powerful man in the country. The couple stated that the previous July, Nicholas Clifton and a gang of armed men ambushed Alice, and the Wests' children Thomas the younger and Alianore, at Malwood in the New Forest. The men raped the unfortunate Alianore West, who, her distressed parents said, was now seriously ill and likely to die as a result of her ordeal. A commission of *oyer et terminer* ('to hear and determine') had been issued on 19 August 1382 naming Nicholas Clifton as the man responsible for raping Alianore at Malwood.

Evidently, Thomas and Alice West were unhappy with the result of this investigation, and were determined to see justice done for the suffering inflicted on their daughter. They therefore called upon the powerful Duke of Lancaster, and Gaunt did see to it that a statute was issued to punish such rapes. However, Nicholas Clifton was pardoned 'for all felonies and rapes with which he is charged' on 14 March 1383, at the request of Richard II's teenage queen, Anne of Bohemia.[17] Some modern writers have speculated that Alianore West staged the whole event to thwart an arranged marriage, and that the situation might have been a voluntary elopement; Alianore later married Clifton, and by 1395 they had a son named Thomas.[18] At any rate, the Wests presented another petition to the parliament held in February 1383, and stated that 'because of their suit, a statute of rapes was made to punish such rapes in future'. A statute 'against the offenders and ravishers of ladies, and the daughters of noblemen and other women' was indeed passed in 1382, though unfortunately it 'withdrew the autonomy of victims to prosecute their attackers without the blessing of their husbands or fathers'.[19]

The examples of Elianore Merton and Katherine Byrom make it painfully apparent that gang rape was not uncommon, and another awful case was that of Joan Gresley, a widow, in the early 1300s. One particularly thuggish and lawless family of the fourteenth-century Midlands was the Swynnertons, a family of at least three brothers who were all knights. Roger Swynnerton, the eldest brother, committed at least two murders; Richard murdered a parson, cut a chaplain's hand off, and beat a man almost to death; and John, while sheriff of Staffordshire, falsely imprisoned a man until he paid a ransom of £20.[20] Richard and John Swynnerton, with other men, 'feloniously captured and abducted' (*felonice ceperunt et rapuerunt*) Joan Gresley from Drakelow near Kidderminster before 25 May 1310, when thirteen men were pardoned for this crime. Seven other men were also involved and were not pardoned on this occasion, and appeared before royal judges sometime between July 1311 and July 1312 and again in June 1324. Joan herself accused about thirty men of breaking into her house, stealing her goods and taking her forty miles to the village of Swynnerton, 'where they detained her for some time'.[21]

Women were vulnerable to attack and assault when they were widows or when their husbands were absent. In 1320, Isabella Gacelyn was abducted from her home in Kenn, Somerset one night while her husband Walter was away. At least sixteen men took part in the abduction, and they placed Isabella on a horse and took her to Newent in the Forest of Dean, over fifty miles away.[22] Olive, widow of John Snard, was 'ravished and aggrieved' by Piers Nevil in Chelveston, Northamptonshire on 20 October 1330.[23] Matilda Fullere, a widow from Shoeburyness in Essex, complained that in April 1383, a chaplain and a parson's servant, with four other men, broke into her house one night. They 'ravished her outside her house' and put her on a horse to abduct her, but when she would not sit still, they took her back inside her home. Matilda was threatened that if she did not marry the parson's servant, whose name appears as 'William Wlips', they would 'immediately kill her'. Then, she said, the men 'compelled her to go to bed with him' and William 'feloniously knew her against her will'. Richard II pardoned Wlips (his name was surely recorded incorrectly) in August 1384.[24] Another chaplain accused of ravishment was John Horewell, and Richard II pardoned him too in October 1398. Horewell was said to have abducted Agnes Beek from her home in Coventry on 17 September 1394 and to have imprisoned her for eight days, though he claimed that he was falsely indicted by the malice of his enemies. Horewell's pardon states that his kidnap and rape of the unfortunate Agnes was done 'against the will of Walter', her husband, not against the will of Agnes herself.[25]

Sometimes the family and friends of rape victims preferred to take matters into their own hands rather than trust the authorities. Margaret Kerevyll of Wiggenhall, Norfolk stated in October 1349 that she had been abducted and 'ravished' by eight people, one of whom, surprisingly, was a woman: Katherine, widow of John Wygenhale. Margaret Kerevyll stated that the eight had come armed to her home, seized her, and imprisoned her in Katherine's house. Margaret's brothers and friends themselves went to Katherine's house and freed her. However, the 'evildoers' continued to plot 'day and night to ravish her again', Margaret said, and to kill her brothers in revenge.[26] In fairness to the Norfolk authorities, 1349 was the year of the first great epidemic of the Black Death, which killed at least a third of the population, so they had much else on their minds, and it is entirely possible that the sheriff and his deputies were among the dead.

On 5 March 1365, William Skynnere (a skinner, i.e. he prepared and sold animal skins) of London entered into a bond with his fellow skinner Richard Palmere 'not to carry away the latter's wife again'. Although this seems like a clear-cut case of abduction – and the 'again' almost gives the situation an element of farce – Richard Palmere had been sent to Newgate prison in London on 2 December 1364 because he 'struck his wife in the breast with a knife'. Palmere was to be imprisoned 'until it was known whether she would die or not'. Palmere's unnamed wife evidently did survive the attack, and William Skynnere's motive in 'carrying her away' was perhaps not to do her harm but to save her from further harm at the hands of her violent husband.[27]

In May 1444, an entry on the Patent Roll records the 'complaint of William Dolbeare of Devon and Margaret late the wife of Thomas Gybbys, deceased, that whereas William agreed with Margaret to marry her at Ayssheberton [Ashburton], and they made oath to celebrate such marriage and the banns were thrice openly published in the parish church of the said town, and afterwards, Margaret being in her place in the said town by night on Tuesday in Passion week last', four named men and eighty others 'ravished the said Margaret, then in bed and lamentably exclaiming and crying, and dragged her from the bed and brought her to a town or place called Foleford and then kept and still keep her'. Two days later, this massive gang lay in wait for William Dolbeare, and 'assaulted and wounded him and took and carried away his goods to the value of £40'. Six months later, Henry VI pardoned John Ferry, John Walssh, William Wynter and John Flour of lying in wait for 'Isabel, daughter of Agnes Hamond' and ravishing her near Framfield in Sussex: another example of gang rape.[28] Richard Lemyng was pardoned in October 1335 for the rape of Elizabeth Tours of Towersey, Buckinghamshire two years earlier, and was again indicted for raping her on a second occasion in 1341. Lemyng protested to Edward III that he had married Elizabeth in 1333 after raping her.[29]

Child Abuse

As Alan Kissane has pointed out, to talk of 'child sexual abuse' in a medieval context is anachronistic, as no such concept existed in any form of medieval law in England.[30] Kissane's research has, however, revealed some horrifying examples of what we would call child abuse and child rape. In 1345/46, eight-year-old Agnes Cloworth was raped by Hugh Outhorp, the local bailiff's sergeant, in Lincoln. Outhorp stole into Agnes's chamber one night and tried to 'contaminate and deflower her', but was unable, owing to her physical immaturity, to penetrate her. Horribly, he cut her wider with his knife and 'violated and ravished her against her will'. Agnes survived this atrocious attack, though barely. Unfortunately for the poor child and her mother Joan, who informed the city authorities what had been done to her daughter, Hugh Outhorp's brother John was one of the two acting bailiffs of Lincoln, and refused to arrest and imprison Hugh. Furthermore, he threatened that he would drive Agnes and Joan out of the city and even out of Lincolnshire altogether.[31]

Caroline Dunn has rightly stated that it is difficult to find cases of child sexual abuse on record, as ages are only rarely given in medieval documents, though she discusses the horrible case of eight-year-old

Alice Chandler and eleven-year-old Joan Seler, raped in London in 1320.[32] Another case of a child abuse victim, also in c. 1320, appears in a petition in French, now in the National Archives. Robert Reppes placed his ten-year-old daughter Eleyne 'with a recluse in Doncaster', but while she was there, the child was abducted by Sir Matthew Bassyngburne, Sir Humphrey Bassyngburne, and other men, and Matthew imprisoned the child in his home and abused her for half a year. Eleyne's father stated that what had been done to his daughter was *encontre son gre e sa volunte*, which either means 'against her social rank and her will' or, more probably, 'against his social rank and his will', meaning her father's. The word used for 'abducted' was *raverunt*, and for what Bassyngburne had done to Eleyne, Robert Reppes used the word *tucha* or 'touched', obviously meant in a sexual sense.[33] Another shocking example (see also Chapter 15 below) is Roger Hales' brutal rape of his own daughter Alice in 1346, which was so appalling that a royal clerk believed, thankfully erroneously, that it had killed her. Alice's age is not known, but her grandfather Sir John Hales was born c. 1306/08 and was still barely forty in 1346, so his son Roger, Alice's father, must have been a young adult and she must have been a young child.[34]

In his research on felonies judged in London in 1321, some of which dated back to the 1270s, Henry Summerson found another distressing case of child abuse. A merchant from Bordeaux, Menald Porte, induced a London brothel-keeper named Agnes Rousse to procure a child for his pleasure, and abused the girl so abominably that he broke her back and she died two weeks later.[35] A case heard before the mayor and aldermen of London in April 1472 most probably also related to the rape or sexual assault of a young girl. John Jordan was 'convicted of a criminal assault upon Margery Scovile, who was under 14 years of age'. Jordan was ordered to pay Margery £40, which would remain in the hands of the chamberlain of London (the city's chief financial officer) until Margery was of full age or married. Within twenty days of his release from prison – the length of the sentence is not given – Jordan was ordered to leave London permanently, and if he did not, would be fined £200 and imprisoned again.[36]

Chapter 15

Incest and Consanguinity

On 16 August 1326, William Melton, Archbishop of York (d. 1340), imposed a penalty on Thomas Raynevill for committing incest with Isabella Folifayt, nun of Hampole Priory in Yorkshire. Thomas was to stand in the church of Hampole, holding a lighted taper of wax in each hand, dressed only in a tunic and bareheaded, and would confess his sin to the congregation. As a further penance, he would be beaten around the nearby parish church of Campsall on two occasions. Melton had already ordered the punishment over two years previously, but Thomas, presumably because of the deep humiliation, had not yet complied.[1] In c. 1323/24, Archbishop Melton imposed a similar penalty on John Overland, a clerk, for incest with Cecilia Salveyn.[2]

Incest had a much broader application in the Middle Ages than it does to us, and it is not necessarily the case that Thomas Raynevill and Isabella Folifayt, and John Overland and Cecilia Salveyn, were brother and sister or uncle and niece, as we might expect. Those who took binding vows of celibacy but subsequently engaged in sexual relations were deemed to have committed incest, such as Isabella Folifayt. Another example was Isabella Westirdale, prioress of Wykeham, in 1444: 'after she had been raised to that office, [she] has been guilty of incest with many men, both within and outside the monastery'.[3]

Furthermore, until 1215 the Church decreed that marriage and sexual relations within seven degrees of kindred were forbidden and incestuous. Unlike today, when the first degree of kindred usually only refers to parents and children, the second degree to siblings, the third to aunts and uncles and so on, the medieval method was simply to count back the number of generations to the last common ancestor. A prohibition on the seventh degree meant therefore that everyone up to and including your sixth cousins was out of bounds sexually and maritally unless dispensed by the pope. As of 1215, anyone with whom you were more distantly related than third cousins (i.e. you had a common set of great-great-grandparents) was permitted. For European royalty, this situation created some difficulties as they were often closely related to each other, though inbreeding among medieval royal families was nowhere near as bad as it became in later centuries. It was rare, though not unheard of, for a royal person between the thirteenth and fifteenth centuries to marry his or her first cousin. Marrying one's second cousin was, however, common: Edward I and Leonor of Castile were second cousins once removed (Leonor was the great-great-granddaughter of Henry II and Eleanor of Aquitaine, while Edward was their great-grandson); Edward II and Isabella of France were also second cousins once removed; Edward III and Philippa of Hainault were second cousins, and Henry IV and Mary de Bohun were second cousins.

Sexual relations with one's spouse's relatives down to their third cousins also counted as incest without a dispensation from the pope. A famous case is Henry VIII, who had an affair with his second wife Anne Boleyn's sister Mary during his first marriage to Katherine of Aragon and required a dispensation before he wed Anne. Thomas Mareschal was excommunicated in 1344 for marrying Isabella Foxle without a papal dispensation, having previously had sex with her sister.[4] Pope Martin V told married couple John Stokker and Joan Blymhyll in 1421 that they were related in the third degree of kindred because John's late first wife Agnes had been related to Joan in the third degree of kindred. Their marriage was, therefore, incestuous as they had not received a dispensation. The same applied to Richard Quinchald and Isabel Amable of Lincolnshire, who married knowing that Richard had previously 'cohabited with' Joan Rokeby, Isabel's second cousin. His sexual relationship with Isabella's kinswoman meant that the couple were related in the third degree, and because they knew that but sought no dispensation and married clandestinely, they were excommunicated in 1392.[5] People who did not know that they were related to their spouse, or to a previous sexual partner of their spouse, were usually treated far more leniently than those who did know but went ahead with their marriage anyway.

Henry Grendon married Elizabeth Peshale in or before 1401 despite knowing that he had previously had relations with a woman related to her in the fourth degree. He eventually confessed to the Bishop of Hereford and received a dispensation from Boniface IX to remain married to Elizabeth.[6] In 1403, the pope ordered the Bishop of Lichfield to issue a dispensation to Sir Henry Hoghton and Joan Radeclyf, of the dioceses of York and Lincoln. They were related in the second degree of kindred on one side of the family and in the third degree on the other, and furthermore, Henry had 'committed fornication with a woman related to Joan in the third degree of kindred'.[7] William Saole and Cecily Caudray of London married in c. 1443, and eight years later William admitted to the Bishop of London that he had had a sexual relationship with Cecily's first cousin, Isabel Morton, before their marriage and had fathered several children with her.[8] John de Warenne, the fifty-eight-year-old Earl of Surrey, famously tried in 1344 to have his childless marriage to Jeanne de Bar annulled on the grounds that before their wedding in 1306, he had 'carnally known' her aunt Mary, Edward I's daughter, a nun at Amesbury Priory. He hoped to persuade Pope Clement VI that he had thereby committed incest for which he had received no dispensation, but his attempt failed.[9] Almost certainly, John's claim was untrue, and he selected Mary because she was closely related to his wife, had been dead for a dozen years and could not gainsay his statement, and had no children to take offence at the claim.

Robert Place of the diocese of York wished to marry his late wife Elizabeth Pudsay's sister in 1437, and, in the interests of being allowed to do so, stated – whether truthfully or not – that Elizabeth had been a leper and that he had never consummated their marriage.[10] William Soper of London carried on an affair with his wife Isabel's cousin Joan Chamberlayn in the 1430s, and 'very often carnally knew her, then a virgin, committing incest' in his marital home. After Isabel's death, William and Joan married *per verba di presenti*, without banns, and the pope dispensed them to remain married and lifted the sentence of excommunication imposed on them by the Bishop of London.[11] Sir Peter Mauley (1281–1348) was absolved by the Archbishop of York in 1313 for committing incest and adultery with his wife's sister Alyna Furnivall, on payment of contributing 100 marks (£66.66) to the fabric of York Minster. Apparently, however, Peter had not learnt his lesson, as in 1323 he was found to have committed adultery with Alice Deyvill and in 1328 with Sara of London.[12] In the early 1200s, an unnamed Oxfordshire man had an affair with his sister-in-law, apparently during his marriage. Pope

Innocent III sent a letter to the prior of Osney Abbey, telling him 'to enjoin a fitting penance on W. [...] who, having married a wife, committed incest and adultery with her sister'. W. claimed that he was too poor to travel to Jerusalem as penance, as ordered, so his wife was told 'not to cohabit with him, and to remain continent during his life'.[13]

Other examples of medieval incest are recorded which would also be classed as incest in modern times, and which, furthermore, seem to represent cases of abuse. Margaret Bothe of the diocese of Coventry and Lichfield took a vow of chastity after the death of her first husband Robert Bothe, though changed her mind and married her second husband Robert Singleton, deeming the breaking of her vow a lesser sin than committing fornication. Singleton, 'overcome by the weakness of the flesh, has, at the instigation of the author of all evil, carnally known' his stepdaughter, Margaret's daughter from her first marriage. Margaret and Robert told Thomas Rotherham, Archbishop of York, that they 'deeply grieve for the said excesses' and for the adultery and incest, and in 1482 Rotherham and Pope Sixtus IV absolved them and enjoined a salutary penance.[14] In 1398, Simon Tychemerch, vicar of Bottesford in Leicestershire and a papal chaplain, was discovered to have 'committed fornication' with his two sisters and had fathered children with both of them.[15] This case, oddly enough, was not called 'incest' in Pope Boniface IX's letter on the matter, and Simon was merely deprived of his vicarage and not otherwise punished.

Sir William Sampson was excommunicated by the Archbishop of York in the early 1300s and imprisoned for committing incest with his daughters Isolde and Clemence, though the archbishop ordered his release on 23 May 1307 on condition that he did penance in Nottingham, Newark and Southwell. Six years later, the Bishop of Durham excommunicated Sir Ralph Neville of Raby (1262–1331), ancestor of the powerful Neville family who became earls of Westmorland at the end of the fourteenth century, for incest with his daughter Anastasia Fauconberg. In addition, Anastasia, whose husband Walter Fauconberg was killed at the Battle of Bannockburn in 1314, and her sister Mary Neville were both accused of adultery with John Lilleford.[16] A particularly horrible case of incest and brutal rape was recorded in July 1346. Roger, son of Sir John Hales, was 'indicted of having ravished and deflowered Alice his own daughter, whereof she died'. Edward III pardoned Hales for the rape, and for another, lesser crime, that of assaulting a couple and their young son after breaking into their house. Just two weeks earlier, Hales had been pardoned for raping another girl or woman, Alice Layton or Laxton.[17] One small consolation is that the clerk who stated that Alice Hales died after her father's violently abusive assault on her was mistaken: she lived long enough to marry two men, Edmund Redesham and George Felbrigg, and was her father's and grandfather's heir. She had no children, however, perhaps a result of the appalling assault on her by her father.[18]

Chapter 16

Same-Sex Relationships

Although nobody in the Middle Ages identified as gay, bi or straight, it is of course beyond all doubt that some people had romantic and/or sexual relationships with members of the same sex. Although it may be that most medieval men were attracted to and had sex with women, and most medieval women were attracted to and had sex with men, 'it would be wrong to attribute to them a consciousness of a heterosexual orientation unless we find evidence for it'. It would also be incorrect to call a medieval person who had relationships with members of the same sex homosexual or gay, as this would be to impose a modern category on them.[1]

In discussing same-sex relations in the Middle Ages, we are hampered by the usual problem, the lack of personal accounts; it is difficult to know how people viewed their own sexuality and sexual desires, and impossible to know for sure how many people engaged in same-sex relations or wished to. As medieval England was a country where men and women, at least at the higher levels of society, were often kept apart, and was a country with a strong military culture where many men spent months or years on end in the company of other men with few if any women around, situational same-sex relations might have been quite common. In the Middle Ages, a sharp distinction was made between procreative and non-procreative sex. Same-sex relations of course fell into the latter category, but so did much opposite-sex sex, and non-procreative intercourse, including same-sex intercourse, was condemned by the Church. Although space does not permit a discussion of the complex meaning of the word 'sodomy' in the Middle Ages, it generally had a wider meaning than it does to us and did not always refer exclusively to male-on-male penetration. James Brundage and Vern L. Bullough have discussed the categories applied by medieval theologians and jurists to sexual acts deemed to be part of *luxuria*, lust or lechery, the deadly 'sin against nature' (*peccatum contra naturam*): *ratione generis* or bestiality; *ratione sexus*, relations with a person having the genitalia of the same sex; and *ratione modi*, having intercourse with a member of the opposite sex but in the wrong orifice, or in a manner that precluded procreation.[2]

A parliament held in Westminster in 1376, late in Edward III's reign, spoke of 'a too horrible vice which should not be named' (*un trop horrible vice qe ne fait pas a nomer*) in relation to merchants and brokers from Lombardy working in England. Modern writers have sometimes assumed this to be a reference to same-sex relations, with the famous words of Lord Alfred Douglas (d. 1945), 'the love that dare not speak its name', in mind. Almost certainly, however, the vice was usury, i.e. charging excessively high rates of interest on loans. A petition by 'the commons of the land' read at the same parliament talked of 'the horrible vice of usury', and stated that the virtue of charity, 'without which nothing might be saved, is almost completely lost' as a result.[3] We should be careful not to impose our own interpretation of what medieval people might have meant by 'horrible vice'.

That being said, it seems that some modern commentators assume that everyone in the past was exclusively attracted to the opposite sex unless we can 100% prove they were not, and it is almost impossible to do so. The only way we can conclusively prove that any two people had intimate relations is if they had children together, and of course, this cannot be the case with people of the same sex. Even Edward II, who had a series of relationships with men from his teens until his forced abdication and imprisonment at the age of forty-two, is said to have probably been 'heterosexual in his tastes'.[4] An abbey annalist in 1326 referred to Edward and his powerful chamberlain and virtual co-ruler Hugh Despenser the Younger as 'the king and his husband', yet it has been suggested that this statement 'should be understood ironically or satirically rather than literally'.[5] Although it is beyond doubt that a person in 1326, almost 700 years before the legalisation of same-sex marriage in the UK, cannot have thought that the two men were literally married (and both of them were married to women), it is hard to imagine that the same rather dismissive attitude would be adopted towards an opposite-sex couple who were not married yet appeared to outsiders to be as intimately close as a married couple. The Flemish chronicler Jean le Bel, who visited England in 1326/27, wrote that Despenser the Younger's penis and testicles were removed during his execution on 24 November 1326 'because he was alleged to be a pervert and a sodomite – above all with the king himself, which was why the king, at his urging, had driven the queen away'.[6] One modern writer has claimed that this statement says nothing about Despenser and Edward's sex life, but refers to Despenser's inferior masculinity and disempowerment as a result of his ignoble behaviour, and on the king's passivity and inability to control him.[7]

All too often, it appears that every piece of evidence for same-sex relations is examined in isolation and dismissed as 'really' meaning something else. If even Edward II, of all people, can be declared to have been exclusively attracted to women, something has gone badly wrong with the burden of proof. There appears to be a double standard: the relationship of Edward's queen Isabella of France and the baron Roger Mortimer between c. 1326 and 1330 is almost always assumed to have been passionately sexual and loving, based on thin evidence, simply because they were a man and a woman. Mortimer is inevitably called the queen's 'lover' in modern books, as though we have webcam footage of the two in bed together. This stands in contrast to most writers' refusal to name Piers Gaveston, Hugh Despenser and the two or three other men with whom Edward II had long-term, intense and serious relationships as his 'lovers'; they are called his 'favourites' or, in older writing, his 'minions'. The only real evidence for Isabella and Mortimer having an affair, except for vague statements in a handful of chronicles, is Jean le Bel's comment that some people thought Isabella was pregnant in 1330 and 'suspected' Mortimer, 'more than anyone', of being the father. Le Bel's statement is taken at face value and as evidence that Isabella probably was pregnant by Roger Mortimer or at least that there were genuine grounds for believing her to be; it is not explained away as really meaning something else, such as an ironic or satirical statement on the queen's inability to control her powerful favourite or on her ignoble behaviour while she ruled her underage son Edward III's kingdom.

Ruth Mazo Karras comments on the 'double standard of evidence', where we 'do not require an eyewitness report of genital contact to state that a given man and woman's attraction to each other was sexual', and we should not require such for a sexual relationship between men or between women either. She has suggested that as many as 10% or

15% of women in northern Europe in the Middle Ages never married. Perhaps at least one reason for this was same-sex attraction, though as Karras points out, we know, sadly, 'excruciatingly little' about medieval women who had sexual relations with other women. As is so often the case, in numerous different cultures and eras, writers were primarily concerned with sexual behaviour only as it related to men and to their choices, and women's actions were fitted into that framework.[8]

One big cultural difference was that in the Middle Ages, people often shared a bed with a member of the same sex without any necessary sexual implications. It showed that you trusted a person not to kill you in your sleep, and was a sign of great favour. Edward IV, for example, invited Henry Beaufort, the staunchly Lancastrian Duke of Somerset, to share his bed after the two men were reconciled in the early 1460s. Despite this favour, however, Beaufort soon turned against the king again. The late historian John Ashdown-Hill claimed that 'it is by no means illogical to deduce' that the two men 'may well have indulged for a time in some kind of sexual intimacy on a regular basis'.[9] Other writers have failed to draw this conclusion and find it unlikely that Edward and Henry were lovers.

Another cultural difference was that medieval men who were most probably not sexually or romantically attracted to other men, or at least not primarily so, were more open about declaring their love for men than is often the case in modern western countries. On hearing that his closest ally and friend Sir Robert Holland had switched sides during the baronial rebellion of 1321/22, Thomas, Earl of Lancaster, groaned, 'How could he find it in his heart to betray me, when I loved him so much?'[10] The ceremony of performing homage to one's liege lord, mostly though not exclusively performed between men, involved kissing on the lips to seal the oath. Edward III, for example, when performing homage as Duke of Aquitaine to Philip VI of France in 1329, kissed Philip on the mouth (*baisa en la bouche*) at the end of the ceremony.[11] Clearly, this kind of kiss had no sexual intent.

As noted above, Edward II had a series of relationships with men, beginning with Piers Gaveston, a young Gascon nobleman placed in his household by his father in or before 1300, when Edward was sixteen or younger. One chronicler stated that 'when the king's son saw him [Gaveston], he fell so much in love that he entered upon an enduring compact with him', and another that 'I do not remember to have heard that one man so loved another'.[12] In 1312, Gaveston was murdered by a group of English barons sick of the king's excessive favouritism towards him. Between early 1315 and 1318/19, Edward appears to have become infatuated with, and to have had relationships with, Sir Roger Damory, Sir Hugh Audley and perhaps Sir William Montacute, and beginning in 1318/19, with his powerful and ruthless chamberlain Hugh Despenser the Younger.

It is the pattern of Edward's behaviour that leads one to conclude that his intense relationships with at least four or five men were almost certainly more than friendship. His sexuality was, however, complex; as noted in Chapter 8 above, in 1324 he left the Tower of London and 'secretly took his pleasure' with a woman, and sometime around 1305/08, fathered an illegitimate son named Adam, who died in 1322. Although the identity of Adam's mother is unknown, Edward must have had a reasonably serious relationship with her to acknowledge paternity of the child. His probable lover Piers Gaveston also fathered an illegitimate child, a daughter whom he named Amie after his sister. It is even possible, peculiarly, that Edward II had an incestuous relationship with his eldest niece Eleanor Despenser, and a chronicler accused him of delighting in 'illicit and sinful sexual intercourse'.[13] This might mean incest, sex with men, both of these, and/or something else entirely.

Edward's great-grandson Richard II formed a very close relationship with Robert de Vere, Earl of Oxford, who, born in 1362, was five years his senior and married the king's cousin Philippa Coucy (b. 1367) in or before 1376. The chronicler Thomas Walsingham wrote that the two men had an 'obscene familiarity' and that Richard 'loved him so much'. Another chronicler, Jean Froissart, said that de Vere's hold over the king was so strong that if Robert said black was white, Richard would not contradict him, and that Robert 'had the sole management of the king'. Froissart also stated that 'the young king was well inclined to follow the advice of the earl, for he loved him with his whole heart'.[14] In 1385 and 1386, Richard gave de Vere the unprecedented titles of Marquis of Dublin and Duke of Ireland, and in late 1387 the young earl fled the country to escape execution at the hands of his baronial enemies. Three chroniclers claimed that Robert de Vere attempted to annul his marriage to Philippa Coucy in the 1380s because he had fallen in love or lust

Same-Sex Relationships

with one of Queen Anne's Bohemian attendants, Agnes Launcekrona, although this does not, of course, preclude the possibility that he was capable of loving men as well. As well as his intense relationship with Robert, Richard II had a very close and loving marriage with his first wife Anne of Bohemia, and was loath to let her leave his side. He grieved terribly when she died at the age of only twenty-eight in 1394, and had the entire palace complex of Sheen, where they had spent much time together, pulled down ten months after Anne's death. As noted in Chapter 6, the couple's childlessness was almost certainly a result of infertility rather than the king's lack of sexual interest in Anne or his desire to live in a chaste marriage.

Chapter 17

Gender Roles and Expectations

Transgender People

Eleanor Rykener was a prostitute arrested in London in 1394 while participating in what was called 'a detestable, unmentionable and ignominious vice' with a man named John Britby, 'lying by a certain stall in Soper's Lane'. When she appeared before the mayor's court, Eleanor turned out to be a man named John Rykener, who was dressed *ut cum muliere*, 'as a woman'. S/he claimed to the court that s/he had been taught how to have sex as a woman by a prostitute named Anna and how to dress as a woman by Elizabeth Brouderer. Rykener stated further that s/he had had plenty of sex both 'as a man' with many nuns and with many other women both married and otherwise, and 'as a woman' with priests and other men in London and in Oxford. In Oxford, Rykener had taken three 'unsuspecting scholars', William Foxlee, John and Walter, into the marshes and had committed the 'abominable vice' with them there. As Isaac Bershady points out, the record states that 'men had sex with [Rykener]', whereas as a man, Rykener had sex with women; here is another example of how medieval gendered language usage paints men as active and women as passive. John/Eleanor Rykener claimed that many of his/her male clients had not noticed that s/he was a man, which seems to reveal that vaginal penetration was perhaps not a common act offered by prostitutes of the era, or at least was not universally expected by their clients.[1]

In London in the second half of the fifteenth century and in the early sixteenth, thirteen women came to the attention of authorities for dressing as men. Margaret Cotton, for example, bought a man's gown from a tailor and wore her male servant's hat, and in 1519 three women all named Margery cut their hair short in what was deemed 'an abomination to the world'. During Edward III's reign, the Leicester chronicler Henry Knighton stated that several dozen well-born women attended a jousting tournament in 'amazing men's clothes' and wearing daggers slung across their stomachs. The disapproving Knighton claimed that the women caused heavy thunderstorms which disrupted the tournament, and were even responsible for the Black Death.[2] In a letter of 1429, Henry VI's uncle John, Duke of Bedford, the child-king's regent of France, referred to Joan of Arc as 'a dissolute woman disguised as a man'.[3] As Ruth Mazo Karras states, in medieval England, and in medieval Europe in general, a strong binary between men and women existed.[4] Men and women who blurred the distinctions were subject to intense social disapproval and even legal action.

Legal Inequality

Medieval England was emphatically not a society where women were legally or socially equal with men. The word most often used for 'husband' in medieval documents was *baron*, and noblewomen always referred to their husbands as *seigneur* or 'lord'. Noblemen called their wives *compaigne*, 'companion' or 'consort', and the language reveals the inequality. Medieval inquisitions and proofs of age talk of 'Adam Brok and Joan his wife, daughter of Thomas Hill' or state that 'John Assheby married Margery, sister of Richard Clete'; women were always identified by reference to their nearest living male relative. Men had control over their wives' actions: in 1391, a man whose name was recorded, peculiarly, as 'George Frwngg' refused to allow his wife Margaret to go on pilgrimage to Santiago de Compostela, as her previous husband Thomas Naunton had ordered her to.[5] Some men openly admitted to hitting and abusing their wives, often for the most tenuous of reasons. While taking part in Robert Burdet's proof of age in Warwickshire in November 1366, John Kent recalled Robert's date of birth in October 1345 because he had been away in Oxfordshire and when he came home, found his wife in their local church with Robert's mother during her purification. Because his wife 'was away on his arrival, he beat her so that she feared for her life'. Jankyn, fifth husband of Chaucer's Wife of Bath, owns a book of tales about the *wikkednesse* of women, and so enrages the Wife by reading aloud from it that she tears out three leaves from it. The furious Jankyn punches her so hard he makes her deaf in one ear. Domestic abuse, however, was sometimes inflicted by women on men: in 1443, John Smith of Bideford in Devon remembered the birth of John Arundell on 9 June 1421 because his wife Lettice beat him that day.[6]

Unlike Henry VIII, medieval English kings did not execute noble or royal women, and none of the victims of the traitor's death from the thirteenth to fifteenth centuries were female; no medieval woman suffered an execution as atrocious as the men who were partially hanged, disembowelled, castrated and finally beheaded before a jeering crowd. Female criminals were, however, hanged, and women could be and were executed for killing their husbands. Under Edward III's Treason Act of 1351, it was deemed petty treason.[7] On the other hand, it was almost impossible to convict a man for the murder of his wife. One tragic example is Alice of Norfolk (b. c. 1324), younger daughter and co-heir of Edward I's son Thomas of Brotherton, Earl of Norfolk, who married the Earl of Salisbury's brother Edward Montacute in or before 1338. In June 1351, Montacute and two of his followers, William Dunch and Thomas, parson of Kelsale, beat Alice so severely that she died of her injuries some months later. Possibly she lapsed into a coma some months after the attack; she was believed to be dead on 14 November 1351 but in fact was still alive, and died sometime before 30 January 1352. The men were never punished, and Alice's cousin Edward III pardoned William Dunch for his involvement in her death on account of his good service in the wars against France. It is probably significant, however, that in November 1351 the king ordered Alice's daughters Maud and Joan Montacute, aged four and two, to be sent to live with their paternal grandmother Elizabeth rather than remaining in their father's custody.[8]

If a woman who was the granddaughter, niece and cousin of kings could be killed with impunity, it is apparent that women of more humble birth stood little chance. Some women accused of murdering their husbands, however, were pardoned, and persuading a powerful person to take an interest in one's case could work wonders. Maud Belhus was imprisoned in the Tower of London in or before April 1304 for murdering her husband Thomas in Bodney, Norfolk, but Edward I pardoned her at the request of his son and heir Edward of Caernarfon, Prince of Wales (later Edward II).[9] Edward of Caernarfon also took a keen interest in the fate of Maud Mortimer, accused of poisoning her husband Hugh in July 1304, and he and his stepmother Queen Marguerite were instrumental in securing Maud's release in 1305.[10] Agnes, the wife of Richard Draycote of Staffordshire, was acquitted of Richard's murder in 1293, and in 1351 Katherine Lakford was acquitted of the murder of her husband John in Bury St Edmunds.[11] Female criminals were spared from execution if they were pregnant, and sometimes the women were subsequently pardoned. In early 1367, Joan Mellere of Suffolk broke into a house and stole 60s in cash, a tunic with a hood and various other items. She was sentenced to death, as thieves in medieval England almost always were, but the sentence was postponed because of her pregnancy. Edward III 'pardoned her the said execution' altogether in July 1371. He also pardoned Beatrice Smyth of Nottinghamshire, convicted of being a 'common thief' in 1376 but found to be pregnant by 'a jury of matrons'.[12]

There were, of course, far fewer female killers in the Middle Ages than male killers, though there are some examples of women killing their lovers. Juliana Aunsel admitted to the murder of her lover Edmund Brekles, a chaplain, in 1324: she stabbed him in the stomach while she was in bed with him, and she and an accomplice, John Maltone, perhaps also her lover, abjured the realm (accepted permanent exile from England). William Mysone, a fishmonger, was killed by his lover Isabel Heyron after a furious row in November 1336 in William's London house. Isabel stabbed William in the heart and he died four days later; she fled and was never caught.[13] A felony specific to women was being a 'common scold'. In 1364, Joan Cotyller, Joan Irlond and Isabel Hemyng were imprisoned as common scolds (recorded in Latin as *communes garulatores*) and brawlers, and in 1375 Alice Shether was also convicted, by a jury of twelve men, of being a common scold.[14]

In medieval England, felons were often sentenced to a period of between one and three hours locked in the pillory. A special pillory for women in London called the *thewe* appears on record from c. 1364 onwards, and was perhaps some kind of ducking-stool. One victim was Alice Salesbury, who in 1373 kidnapped a child named Margaret Oxewyk and stripped her to increase her takings while begging (passersby would feel more sympathy for a woman with a naked child). In the 1360s and 1370s, several women were condemned to the *thewe* for coating the bottom of a quart measure for ale with pitch so that customers 'lost a third of its contents', and another for selling bad fish. The oddly-named Albredala Veyse was imprisoned in 1364 after claiming publicly, but wrongly, that her neighbour Rose Whytcherche had been put on the *thewe* for 'selling ale contrary to regulations'. Albredala was released after promising to behave herself and to 'bridle her tongue'.[15]

In 1406, the mayor and aldermen of London dealt with a complaint that female prisoners in Newgate (the city's largest and most notorious prison) were uncomfortably detained in a very small cell. When the women needed to use the privy, they had to pass through a much larger cell called *Bocardo* where men were held, 'to their great shame and hurt'. The solution was to build a new stone tower just to the south of the prison solely for women, with its own facilities. A series of ordinances regarding the treatment of prisoners in Newgate, issued in early 1431, makes apparent that women now had their own 'large chamber near the hall on the south side' of the prison.[16]

Property and Female Merchants

Married women's lands and goods officially belonged to their husbands, and in almost all circumstances it was only as widows that women could make wills and dispose of their own belongings. One exception was the Queen of England, who, though married, owned her lands as a 'sole woman', but still required the king's permission to make a will. Queen Isabella received this permission from her husband Edward II on 20 October 1312 while she was heavily pregnant with their first child, Edward III (born twenty-four days later).[17] Some female merchants in London were also given the status of *feme sole* or sole woman: 'If a *feme covert*, the wife of a freeman, trades by herself in a trade, with which her husband does not intermeddle, she may sue and be sued as a *feme sole*'.[18] In 1381, Alice atte Wode, as a sole woman, undertook to 'provide for her father competently, according to his rank, in food, clothing, bed, shoes and other necessaries, and to give him 14d a week to spend as he liked'.[19]

Many professions were restricted and were not open to women, though in 1310 Robert Newcomen completed a ten-year apprenticeship in London with 'Henry the Surgeon and Katherine, wife of the same'.[20] It appears that in the early 1300s, a London woman was medically and surgically trained. In 1390, four male master surgeons of London were sworn in to make 'faithful scrutiny' of 'others, both men and women, undertaking cures, or practising the art of surgery'.[21] In medieval England, women often made a living by brewing ale, and were called brewsters; men who brewed ale were brewers. Many medieval job titles had a -ster(e) ending which showed that the person was female, because, as many other European languages were and are, Middle English was gendered. Examples are: *frutere* and *frutestere* (male and female fruit-sellers), *callere* and *callestere* (male and female makers or sellers of headdresses), *bredmongere* and *bredmongestere* (male and female bread-sellers), *bakstere* (female baker), *rokstere* (a woman or girl who rocked an infant's cradle), *cambestere* (a woman who made or sold combs), *hokstere* or *huckestere* (hawker or peddler), *tappestere* (tavern-keeper), *spinstere*, a female spinner, and *web(be)stere*, a female *webbe* or weaver. Some of these words survive in the twenty-first century as family names, such as Webster, Brewster and Baxter (*bakstere*), or as modern words with a different meaning: 'huckster' has pejorative connotations which it did not have in the Middle Ages and no longer refers solely to women, and 'spinster' no longer means a female spinner and also has deeply pejorative connotations.

Primogeniture and Valuing Boys

Medieval inheritance law favoured men, and lands held by tenants in chief passed preferentially to a male heir. Primogeniture, the system where the eldest son inherited everything, did not apply to female heirs, who, in the absence of a male heir, inherited equal shares of an estate. This gave landowners a strong motivation to have sons, to avoid their lands being broken up after their deaths. After Fulk Fitzwarin was born in Wantage, Berkshire (now Oxfordshire) on 14 September 1251, 'the father and friends were much congratulated, because all his other children were girls'. Joan Eglesfeld was born in Penrith, Cumberland on 3 February 1355. Her father John grumbled to a man he met in the market that the birth 'displeased him ... because he would have been glad of a son' (as it turned out, he had no son or other daughter, and Joan was his heir).[22] William Ferrers, Earl of Derby (d. 1254), had seven daughters with his first wife Sybil Marshal, and faced the prospect of his earldom being divided into seven parts after his death. However, he had two sons (and three more daughters) with his second wife Margaret Quency, and the birth of their first son Robert in c. 1239 immediately disinherited Robert's older half-sisters from any share in the Ferrers lands. Sybil was herself one of the five daughters of William Marshal, Earl of Pembroke (d. 1219), and after William's five sons all died without offspring, his daughters' dozens of children and grandchildren, including Sybil's seven daughters and their children, inherited equal portions of the estate.

Much evidence exists, however, to show that where the descent of property was not bound to pass to male heirs preferentially, many men left their houses, as well as money, jewellery, clothes, household vessels and other items, to their sons and daughters in equal portions. In 1307, Laurence Lillebourne ordered his tenement in London to be sold and the proceeds to be divided equally among his children John, Peter and Isabel. In 1316/17, John Dittone left jewels, linen cloth, beds and chattels to his daughter Isabel, unspecified other 'chattels' to his daughter Joan, and sums of money to his sons Thomas and Richard and the unborn child his wife Isabel was carrying. At the same time, the vintner Stephen Feryng left his tenement to his children Robert, Henry and Isabel in equal parts. John of Paris left his tenements to his sons John, Roger and Stephen and his daughters Maud, Denise and Agnes in his will dated 20 July 1321, and a few days later, Roger of Paris, a mercer, requested that after his death, his corner shop in St Pancras should be sold. The proceeds were to be distributed not only among his own two sons and two daughters, Simon, John, Maud and Joan, but to his stepdaughter Alice, his wife Margaret's daughter from a previous marriage. Roger Waltham divided his goods, houses and wharf equally among his six daughters and two sons in July 1342, and in April 1349, Simon Brunnesford left his son William £5, but gave £20 to each of his four daughters. In his 1349 will, William Thorneye left a parcel of land called *Personbroderove* near Wisbech, Cambridgeshire to five women: Alice Saleman, Joan Rolle and Maud Bageys, daughters of his late sister Lettice Bageneye, and Alice and Joan's daughters, both named Margery, William's great-nieces. Henry Baundeney, an illuminator of Lincoln, left almost all his property to his daughter Beatrice rather than his son Osbert in 1296.[23]

Sex Ratios

Sandy Bardsley has suggested that in late medieval England, there were as many as 110 or 115 men for every 100 women, and that fewer females lived into adulthood and even when they did, often died younger than their husbands and brothers. Research shows that around the middle of the thirteenth century, the proportion of women began to decline, stabilised for a while after the pandemics of the Black Death in the fourteenth century, and fell again in the fifteenth.[24] One contemporary chronicler, writing in Middle English, claimed that the second pandemic of plague in England in 1361/62 killed more men than women, and if this is true, it might go some way to explaining the stabilised sex ratio. Supposedly, the victims' widows, 'out of governance' after their husbands' deaths, married 'lewd and simple men' instead, and 'coupled ... with them that were of low degree and little reputation'.[25] In her work on orphans in medieval London, Barbara Hanawalt notes that girls were less likely to survive childhood than boys, and puts the disparity at an average of a 10% shortfall in girls over the period from 1309 to 1497. Both Bardsley and Hanawalt note that the reasons for the discrepancy are complex, though Hanawalt suggests that care and nurturing in childhood, rather than female infanticide, might be to blame, and that 'male children were given better care because they had a higher social value'.[26]

Valued Women

The wish to have sons and to prevent an inheritance being broken up among a number of female heirs, and the undeniable fact that boys were often valued more than girls, did not, however, necessarily mean that men did not love their daughters. They and their contemporaries often expressed their joy at the birth of a girl. Edward I's grandson Thomas Monthermer (1301–40) celebrated the birth of his daughter and heir Margaret in Stokenham, Devon in October 1329 by hunting deer in his park there. Katherine Plaunke was born on 6 January 1341 in Befcote, Staffordshire, the eldest of her parents' three daughters, and two local men saw her being carried to her baptism and back home again 'with singing and a great concourse of people praising God for her birth'. When Mary Barnak was born in Shelfanger, Norfolk on 8 September 1406 as the third child and second daughter of her parents, she was baptised 'amid great rejoicing'. Joan Wybbury was born in Cockington, Devon on 10 August 1424, and a servant of her maternal grandfather John Gorgeys walked to nearby Torre Abbey, whose abbot was to be Joan's godfather, to inform the monks. On hearing the news, 'a monk joyfully said 'Come to the church and give thanks to Almighty God!"[27]

There is much evidence for men loving their wives, daughters and sisters dearly. William Quyntyn married his wife Thephania in

Cambridgeshire sometime in 1283, but she died not long afterwards in November 1284, whereupon he 'was almost mad with grief'. After John Scolmayster married his wife Christine on the morning of 18 January 1403, he went back to the same church some hours later to attend a baptism. When he returned home, he found Christine dead, and talked many years later of the 'bitterness of his distressed soul'. In 1329, John Coleman of Essex recalled the death of his 'beloved daughter' Margaret in November 1304, and Sir Peter Thornton of the diocese of Lichfield, distressed at the illness of his wife Lucy in 1333, made a vow to visit Jerusalem in order to pray that Lucy would recover. John Croft of Herefordshire remembered in 1360 how his 'beloved sister' Margaret Croft had died on 3 February 1338, and how he had his village priest enter her obit in the church missal and sometimes, decades later, still looked at it.[28]

The curiously named Walkelina Elyot died in infancy in Ashton, Devon on 18 January 1403 (on the same day and in the same village as Christine Scolmayster). Her father William blamed her death on the 'lack of care' of Walkelina's nurse, who allowed the little girl to die of thirst in her cradle. William walked to his local church to ask the parson to say divine services for his daughter's soul on the day of her death, and twenty-two years later said sadly that 'the memory of this misfortune has never left him'.[29] A moving poem called *Pearl*, written in the north-west of England in the late fourteenth century, begins with the narrator grieving for his dead infant daughter, his 'pearl', buried in his garden. He goes to lie on her grave, falls asleep, and has a vivid dream about meeting and talking to her as a little Queen of Heaven. They are separated by a river, and when the narrator tries to cross, he wakes, and finds himself still lying on his daughter's grave.

Abbreviations

CCR	Calendar of Close Rolls
CIM	Calendar of Inquisitions Miscellaneous
CIPM	Calendar of Inquisitions Post Mortem
Coroner	Calendar of Coroners Rolls of the City of London
CPL	Calendar of Papal Registers Relating to Great Britain and Ireland: Papal Letters
CPR	Calendar of Patent Rolls
EMCR	Calendar of Early Mayor's Court Rolls, 1298–1307
LBA	Calendar of Letter-Books of the City of London, Letter-Book A, 1275–1298
LBB	Letter-Books of the City of London, Letter-Book B, 1275–1312
LBC	Letter-Book C, 1291–1309
LBD	1309–1314
LBE	1314–1337
LBF	1337–1352
LBG	1352–1374
LBH	1375–1399
LBI	1400–1422
LBK	1422–1457
LBL	1460–1496
MLL	Memorials of London and London Life in the 13th, 14th and 15th Centuries

PP	Petitions to the Pope 1342–1419
PROME	Parliament Rolls of Medieval England
SAL MS 122	Society of Antiquaries of London, Manuscript no. 122
SPMR	Calendar of Select Plea and Memoranda Rolls of the City of London; vol. 1: 1323–64; vol. 2: 1364–81; vol. 3: 1381–1412
Statutes	Statutes of the Realm, vols. 1 and 2
TNA	The National Archives (BCM: Berkeley Castle Muniments; DL: Duchy of Lancaster; E: Exchequer; SC: Special Collections)
Wills, part 1	Calendar of Wills Proved and Enrolled, part 1, 1258–1358
Wills, part 2	Calendar of Wills Proved and Enrolled, part 2, 1358–1688

Notes

Chapter 1: Appearance

1. Bigelow, 'Bohun Wills', 635, 641.
2. *Coroner*, 147–8; *MLL*, 109; *SPMR*, vol. 2, 154–6.
3. http://www.medievalgenealogy.org.uk/inquests/abstracts_106.shtml (Abstracts of Coroners' Inquests in Northamptonshire, accessed 23 April 2021); *Coroner*, 59, 127, 190, 221, 257.
4. Geaman, 'Struggle to Conceive', 229.
5. *The Trotula*, ed. Green, 112–19.
6. See https://www.gutenberg.org/files/24790/24790-h/nurture.html lines 975 on, accessed 14 April 2021; *The Babees' Book*, ed. Rickert and Naylor, 34–5. Edward II's servants paid 21d in London in 1325 for pink and white roses to make rose-water: SAL MS 122, 6, 9.
7. Johnstone, 'Wardrobe and Household of Henry', 390, 396–7, 402; Woolgar, *Great Household*, 166–70.
8. Mortimer, *Time Traveller's Guide*, 196; Woolgar, *Senses in Late Medieval England*, 135–6.
9. Mathew, *Court of Richard II*, 32–4.
10. *Livre de Seyntz Medicines*, ed. Arnould, 194, 202–3; Woolgar, *Great Household*, 167–8; *Trotula*, ed. Green, 113.
11. For the *Lavenderebrigge*, see e.g. *Coroner*, 100; http://www.medievalgenealogy.org.uk/inquests/abstracts_107.shtml, accessed 23 April 2021.
12. *MLL*, 648.
13. Tout, *Place of the Reign*, 279; Myers, *Household of Edward IV*, 196–7.
14. Woolgar, *Senses*, 128–9, 132–3, 166; Mortimer, *Time Traveller*, 194–6.
15. *Seyntz Medicines*, ed. Arnould, 13–14, 47–9.

16. *Oxford Dictionary of National Biography*.
17. *Trotula*, 112; https://www.historyextra.com/period/medieval/did-medieval-people-take-baths-why-they-were-cleaner-than-we-think-middle-ages-hygiene-handwash-washing-cleanliness-coronavirus-plague-covid, accessed 19 May 2021, for Gilbert.
18. *The Book of the Duchess*, lines 948–59; http://www.librarius.com/duchessfs.htm, accessed 23 May 2021.
19. https://sites.fas.harvard.edu/~chaucer/teachslf/milt-par.htm, line 3234, accessed 14 April 2021.
20. Rees, *Caerphilly Castle*, 109–21.
21. Rhodes, 'Inventory of the Jewels', 518–21; Mortimer, *Time Traveller*, 105–6.
22. *John of Gaunt's Register 1371–75*, nos. 931, 1133, 1343.
23. *Trotula*, 115–16.
24. SAL MS 122, 66.
25. *EMCR*, 92; *LBC*, 79; TNA E 101/380/4.
26. Mortimer, *Time Traveller*, 103–4.
27. SAL MS 122, 9, 42–3, 69, 79, 86.
28. *CPR 1327–30*, 98–9; *CPR 1330–34*, 363.
29. *Book of Chivalry*, ed. Kaeuper and Kennedy, 191–3.
30. *LBA*, 220; *LBH*, 176; *MLL*, 267, 458.

Chapter 2: Marriage (1)

1. *SPMR*, vol. 1, 153.
2. Ormrod, 'Edward III and his Family', 410 note 46.
3. *CIPM 1361–65*, no. 118; *Knighton's Chronicle*, ed. Martin, 30; TNA DL 27/36; *CPR 1338–40*, 213; *CPR 1343–45*, 366.
4. *CIPM 1347–52*, no. 56; *CIPM 1370–73*, no. 210; *CPR 1350–54*, 50, 67.
5. Baldwin, *Elizabeth Woodville*, 10; *CIPM 1361–65*, no. 550.
6. For more information on the courtesy of England, see also Chapter 3 below. John Beaufort's and his uncle Cardinal Beaufort's inquisitions post mortem, naming Margaret as heir, are in *CIPM 1442–47*, nos. 178–94, 582.
7. *CPL 1431–47*, 579; *CPL 1447–55*, 607–8.
8. *CChR 1257–1300*, 427; *CIPM 1347–52*, no. 107; Maddicott, *Thomas of Lancaster*, 3.

Notes

9. *CPR 1266–72*, 323; *CPL 1198–1304*, 450.
10. *CPL 1305–41*, 527.
11. *Wills*, part 1, 423, 467–8; *MLL*, 248–9, 310; *LBD*, 183–4; *LBF*, 203; *LBG*, 10, 91, 141, 317; *LBH*, 165.
12. *CIPM 1317–27*, no. 696; *CIPM 1327–36*, no. 229; *Wills*, part 1, 238, 352.
13. *CIPM 1384–92*, no. 342.
14. *CIPM 1365–69*, no. 189; *CIPM 1384–92*, no. 77; *CIPM 1392–99*, no. 275; *CIPM 1405–13*, no. 901; *CIPM 1413–18*, no. 270; see also my book *Living in Medieval England: The Turbulent Year of 1326*, 147–8.
15. *CIPM 1399–1405*, no. 858.
16. *LBE*, 47–8; *Wills*, part 1, 257, 277.
17. *LBG*, 181, 213; *LBH*, 52, 357–60; *Wills*, part 2, 79, 81; *CIPM 1235–72*, no. 202.
18. *John of Gaunt's Register 1379–83*, no. 463; *CIPM 1370–73*, no. 148; *CIPM 1384–92*, nos. 12, 13, 20.
19. *CPR 1354–58*, 595; Feet of Fines, CP 25/1/288/47, no. 637 (available on medievalgenealogy.org.uk); *CIPM 1361–65*, no. 592; *CIPM 1377–84*, nos. 179–89; *CFR 1413–22*, 166–7.
20. *CIPM 1392–99*, nos. 421–22, 1093; *CIPM 1399–1405*, nos. 31–38; *CIPM 1413–18*, nos. 190–94; *CIPM 1418–22*, nos. 443–6; *CFR 1391–99*, 254; *CPR 1396–99*, 516.
21. *CIPM 1413–18*, no. 701; *CIPM 1427–32*, no. 412.
22. *LBL*, 85, 143.
23. *Prologe of the Wyves Tale of Bathe*, line 6.
24. *SPMR*, vol. 3, 152–3; *CIPM 1336–46*, no. 65; *Wills*, part 1, 45, 75.
25. *CIPM 1352–60*, no. 641; *CIPM 1384–92*, no. 78.
26. *CIPM 1432–37*, no. 26; *CPL 1342–62*, 456.
27. *CIPM 1327–36*, no. 698; *CIPM 1377–84*, no. 659; *CIPM 1405–13*, nos. 781, 786.
28. Wodderspoon, *Memorials of the Ancient Town*, 248.
29. *CIPM 1370–73*, no. 313. John was to claim years later that he had never truly married Aubrey; see below.
30. *CIPM 1272–91*, no. 819.
31. *Manuale et Processionale*, p. xvi, Appendix p. 19*.
32. *MLL*, 561–2, 571; *CLI*, 72, 85; *SPMR*, vol. 3, 291; *CIM 1219–1307*, nos. 359, 2099, 2283.
33. *CIPM 1432–37*, no. 272.

34. Wade Labarge, *Mistress, Maids and Men*, 140, 143–4.
35. Smyth, *Lives of the Berkeleys*, vol. 2, 30.
36. *CIPM 1291–1300*, no. 629; *CIPM 1307–17*, no. 153; *CIPM 1413–18*, no. 264; *CIPM 1422–27*, nos. 359, 530.
37. https://www.thoughtco.com/weddings-and-hygiene-1788715, accessed 31 March 2021.
38. *CIPM 1405–13*, nos. 671, 780; *CIPM 1418–22*, no. 758; *CIPM 1427–32*, no. 417; *CIPM 1432–37*, no. 267; *CIPM 1437–42*, nos. 527, 613, 724; *CIPM 1442–47*, nos. 196, 241, etc.
39. Mortimer, *Fears of Henry IV*, 260.
40. See https://pages.uoregon.edu/dluebke/Reformations441/441Marriage Law.html, accessed 2 April 2021.
41. Sturcken, 'Unconsummated Marriage', 185–201; Joseph, 'Dynastic Marriage in England, Castile and Aragon', 26.
42. See https://pages.uoregon.edu/dluebke/Reformations441/441Marriage Law.html, accessed 2 April 2021.
43. Donahue, *Law, Marriage and Society*, 135–6; *CIPM 1235–72*, no. 303.
44. Santos Silva, 'Portuguese Household of an English Queen', 272.

Chapter 3: Marriage (2)

1. *CPL 1398–1404*, 609; *CPL 1427–47*, 601; *CFR 1422–30*, 32; *CPR 1422–29*, 136. Margery Despenser and Roger Wentworth were the great-grandparents of Margery Wentworth (*c.* 1478–1550), who married Sir John Seymour of Wolf Hall in 1494 and whose daughter Jane Seymour became Henry VIII's third queen in 1536.
2. Cited in McCarthy, *Medieval Marriage*, 93.
3. *CPL 1305–41*, 274; *CPL 1427–47*, 267–8, 518–19.
4. *Statutes*, vol. 1, 302.
5. *CPR 1361–64*, 408; *CPR 1441–46*, 163.
6. *CPL 1458–71*, 471.
7. Brundage, *Law, Sex*, 478; Bellamy, *Criminal Law and Society*, 116.
8. *CPL 1404–15*, 415; *CPR 1377–81*, 101, 232.
9. *CIPM 1272–91*, no. 766; *CPR 1281–92*, 335; *CPR 1422–29*, 111.
10. *CCR 1296–1302*, 145, 226; *CCR 1354–60*, 367.
11. *CFR 1307–19*, 26; *CCR 1307–13*, 76. Margaret and Edmund's eldest son Ralph Stafford (1301–72) was the first Earl of Stafford. Edmund was born on 15 July 1273: *CIPM 1291–1300*, no. 202.

Notes

12. *CPR 1367–70*, 146. Joan died a year later, probably only eighteen years old: *CIPM 1365–69*, no. 406.
13. *CPR 1324–27*, 267; *CPR 1334–38*, 241; *CPR 1343–45*, 350. Margaret and Hereford discovered in 1331 that they were related in the fourth degree, and 'ceased to live together' until the matter was resolved: *CPL 1305–41*, 349.
14. *CPR 1401–05*, 242; *Royal and Historical Letters During the Reign*, vol. 2, 87–102.
15. *CPR 1313–17*, 553; *CPR 1422–29*, 271–2, 543; *CIPM 1370–73*, no. 223; *CIM 1348–77*, no. 126; *CCR 1349–54*, 603; *CIPM 1352–60*, no. 124; *CIPM 1300–07*, no. 56; *CCR 1302–7*, 24.
16. *CCR 1279–88*, 462; TNA SC 1/10/109, E 159/60, membrane 14d; Prestwich, 'Royal Patronage Under Edward I', 44.
17. *CFR 1307–19*, 380, 388, 394; *CPR 1317–21*, 387, 582.
18. *CPL 1427–47*, 514–15; *CPR 1436–41*, 160.
19. *CPR 1409–13*, 90.
20. *CPR 1313–17*, 535; *Complete Peerage*, vol. 5, 584–5; *CIPM 1317–27*, no. 54.
21. *CPR 1307–13*, 409–10, 560; *CIPM 1307–17*, nos. 352, 565; *CIPM 1317–27*, nos. 192, 274.
22. *CPR 1381–85*, 353; *CPR 1391–96*, 8; *CPR 1408–13*, 307.
23. *CIPM 1317–27*, no. 618; *CIPM 1327–36*, no. 276; *CFR 1319–27*, 357–8; *CCR 1330–33*, 162.
24. *CIM 1219–1307*, no. 1218; *CIPM 1235–72*, no. 414; *CIPM 1384–92*, no. 6; *CIPM 1413–18*, no. 847; *LBG*, 163–4; *LBH*, 357–60.
25. *CIPM 1422–27*, nos. 813, 831.
26. *CPR 1381–85*, 229, 236; *CPR 1389–92*, 16; *CIPM 1374–77*, no. 105; *CIPM 1377–84*, nos. 1022–27.
27. *CPL 1305–41*, 209.
28. *CIPM 1291–1300*, no. 620.
29. *CCR 1313–18*, 74–5, 393; *CPR 1307–13*, 380; *CFR 1307–19*, 120; *CIPM 1307–17*, no. 346.
30. *CIPM 1307–17*, no. 151; *CPR 1307–13*, 273.
31. *SPMR*, vol. 3, 155; *Wills*, part 2, 237; *Calendar to the Feet of Fines for London and Middlesex*, vol. 1, Henry IV no. 33.
32. *CIPM 1327–36*, no. 169; *CIPM 1405–13*, nos. 997, 1005.
33. *Wills*, part 1, 354–5; *LBE*, 250, 256.
34. Cited in Peltzer, 'Marriages of the English Earls', 73–4.

35. *CFR 1399–1405*, 130–1; *CCR 1399–1402*, 381–3; *CIPM 1399–1405*, nos. 908–27. Robert was in Thomas Mowbray's household by August 1390: *CIPM 1405–13*, no. 336.
36. *CPR 1350–54*, 199; *CFR 1347–56*, 317; *CFR 1356–68*, 33.

Chapter 4: Marriage (3)

1. *Book of Chivalry*, ed. Kaeuper and Kennedy, 171–3.
2. *CPR 1324–27*, 153; *CPR 1327–30*, 325.
3. *Complete Peerage*, vol. 12B, 753–4; *CPR 1247–58*, 172.
4. *Wills*, part 1, 323; *LBD*, 184–6.
5. *Wills,* part 1, 455–6; *London Possessory Assizes*, no. 13; *CPR 1358–61*, 101; Feet of Fines, Oxfordshire, CP 25/1/190/21, no. 40, available on medievalgenealogy.org.uk.
6. TNA BCM/D/1/1/9, BCM/D/1/1/11; *CPL 1342–62*, 327; *CIPM 1352–60*, no. 564.
7. *CIPM 1405–13*, nos. 604–11; *Complete Peerage*, vol. 10, 661–2; *Testamenta Vetusta*, vol. 1, 92–3.
8. *Wills*, part 1, 263, 268–9, 506, 515–16, 518, 634.
9. *Wills*, part 2, 19–20, 77, 102–3, 278–9; *LBG*, 122; *CIPM 1307–17*, no. 68.
10. *Wills*, part 2, 16, 75, 161–2, 448–9, 451; *SPMR*, vol. 3, 103.
11. *CIPM 1235–72*, no. 389; *CIPM 1272–91*, no. 477; *CCR 1302–7*, 405; *PP*, 133–4.
12. *SPMR*, vol. 3, 151.
13. Morris, *The Bigod Earls*, 125.
14. *CIPM 1291–1300*, no. 391; *CFR 1272–1307*, 391.

Chapter 5: Marriage (4)

1. *CPR 1334–38*, 283, 298.
2. *CIPM 1307–17*, no. 131.
3. *CPR 1266–72*, 520–21; *CCR 1268–72*, 294–5. Giffard was the boy who married Aubrey Camville in 1241 when they were both children, and later repudiated the marriage.
4. *CIPM 1291–1300*, no. 544; *CIPM 1327–36*, no. 180. Katherine Giffard, married to Nicholas Audley, was said to be twenty-seven in 1299, while her sisters Eleanor and Maud were twenty-four and

twenty-two. Then again, Maud Clifford's daughter from her first marriage, Margaret, Countess of Lincoln, was said to be thirty in 1299 when in fact she was in her mid-forties. Giffard's heir was his son from his third marriage, John the younger, born in June 1287 when Giffard was about fifty-five.

5. TNA SC 8/64/3163; *CPR 1334–38*, 282, 319; *CFR 1327–37*, p. 473; *CPR 1334–38*, 379–80, 398; *CCR 1333–37*, 554, 561–2, 564, 722, 726, 736; *CCR 1337–39*, 18–20, 25; *Anonimalle Chronicle 1333–81*, ed. Galbraith, 8.
6. Donahue, *Law, Marriage and Society*, 169–71.
7. McSheffrey and Pope, 'Ravishment, Legal Narratives', 820–2.
8. *SPMR*, vol. 2, 247. South Mimms is now in Hertfordshire.
9. *Wills*, part 2, 19–20, *LBG*, 122.
10. *SPMR*, vol. 3, 18, 22–3.
11. *Wills*, 332; *LBE*, 47, 229, 266–7.
12. *CPR 1313–17*, 320, 409, 506, 580–1.
13. *CIM 1308–48*, no. 1582; *CIPM 1336–46*, no. 98; *CCR 1337–39*, 82.
14. *CCR 1330–33*, 90–1, 93–4; *Life-Records of Chaucer*, ix; TNA SC 8/169/8432.
15. TNA SC 8/152/7598; *CPR 1307–13*, 384.
16. *Statutes*, vol. 1, 88–9.
17. *CPR 1313–17*, 422; *CFR 1307–19*, 266; *CCR 1323–27*, 440–41.
18. *CIPM 1235–72*, nos. 124, 875; *CIPM 1370–73*, no. 313.
19. *Oxford Dictionary of National Biography*.
20. *CPR 1327–30*, 23; *CPL 1342–62*, 381, 391; *CPR 1354–58*, 93, 325; *CCR 1354–60*, 27.
21. *CPL 1342–62*, 164, 176, 188; *PP*, 75, 81, 99.
22. *PP*, 75, 81, 99; *CPL 1342–62*, 164, 188, 254; *CPL 1362–1404*, 74.
23. Tompkins, 'Mary Percy and John de Southeray', 133–56.
24. *CPL 1427–47*, 545; *CPL 1471–84*, 503–4.
25. TNA SC 8/18/889; *PROME*, October 1378 parliament; *CPR 1377–81*, 260, 299, 301, 303, 309, 311, 374, 530; *CCR 1374–77*, 158; *CCR 1377–81*, 149, 204, 220, 222–3, 227–8; *CCR 1381–85*, 34, 389; *CPR 1396–99*, 544; *CIPM 1361–65*, no. 565; *CIPM 1374–77*, nos. 180, 274; *CIPM 1392–99*, nos. 508–12; *CIPM 1422–27*, nos. 760–1; *Excerpta Historica*, ed. Bentley, 424–6.
26. Butler, *Language of Abuse*, 131.
27. Donahue, *Law, Marriage and Society*, 139–40.

28. McCarthy, *Medieval Marriage*, 96; http://www.medievalgenealogy.org.uk/inquests/abstracts_107.shtml, accessed 23 April 2021.
29. *CPL 1398–1404*, 320; *CPL 1455–64*, 188–9, 319; *CPL 1471–84*, 515.
30. *SPMR*, vol. 2, 117, 173 (Joan Coutenhale); https://inews.co.uk/light-relief/offbeat/throwback-thursday-medievalists-take-impotence-tests-79765, accessed 10 May 2021 (Chobham quotation); Kane, *Impotence and Virginity*, 9–10 (Alice Russell and Joan Gilbert).
31. *SPMR*, vol. 3, 151–3, 185; *CPR 1381–85*, 164.
32. *EMCR*, 230; *LBB*, 168; *Wills*, part 1, 76, 148.
33. *Statutes*, vol. 1, 87, and see also Chapters 4 and 7.
34. Butler, 'Runaway Wives', 340.
35. *EMCR*, 230.

Chapter 6: Sexual Pleasure and Relationships (1)

1. Cited and translated in Niebrzydowski, *Bonoure and Buxum*, 100–01.
2. Brundage and Bullough, *Handbook of Medieval Sexuality*, 84–5; Cadden, *Meanings of Sex Difference*, 86, 97–8, 142–4; Niebrzydowski, *Bonoure and Buxum*, 100; Mortimer, *Time Traveller*, 55.
3. Cited in Leyser, *Medieval Women: A Social History*, 96.
4. *The Trotula*, ed. Green, 91.
5. *Book of Holy Medicines*, ed. Batt, 122, 229–30; *Livre de Seyntz Medicines*, ed. Arnould, 78, 179.
6. *Seyntz Medicines*, 66–7, 72, 77.
7. *Prologe of the Wyves Tale of Bathe*, lines 565, 597–9.
8. Schaus, *Women and Gender*, 755; Kane, *Impotence and Virginity*, 12.
9. *CPL 1342–62*, 167, 173; *CPL 1471–84*, 309–10.
10. Karras, *Sexuality in Medieval Europe*, p. 38; *Flores Historiarum*, vol. 3, ed. Luard, 70; quotation from Magna Carta taken from https://www.nationalarchives.gov.uk/education/resources/magna-carta/magna-carta-1225-westminster, accessed 1 April 2021.
11. TNA SC 1/63/150; *CPL 1342–62*, 113.
12. *CPL 1305–41*, 544.
13. *CPL 1398–1404*, 536; *CPL 1447–55*, 55.
14. *CPL 1305–41*, 544; *CPL 1471–84*, 835–6.

15. *CPR 1350–54*, 336. Kendale was probably a younger son of Sir Robert Kendale (d. 1330), whose heir was his eldest son Edward (*c.* 1309–73). Margaret died on 31 October 1373, and her husband Hamo was a brother of Fulk Lestrange of Cheswardine: *CIPM 1374–77*, no. 77.
16. *CPL 1447–55*, 212.
17. *CPR 1381–85*, 192, 263; Geaman, 'Personal Letter', 1086–94; Geaman, 'Struggle to Conceive', 10–12.
18. *London Possessory Assizes*, nos. 28, 30; *Wills*, part 1, 353, 378.
19. *Wills*, part 1, 186–7, 285; Wills, part 2, 521–2.

Chapter 7: Sexual Pleasure and Relationships (2)

1. *Book of Chivalry*, ed. Kaeuper and Kennedy, 119–23.
2. All the cases below are taken from *LBI*, 273–87, unless otherwise stated.
3. *SPMR*, vol. 3, 148 (which also gives the details about John Norhampton cited in Walsingham); *LBH*, 176, 189.
4. *LBH*, 339.
5. *CPL 1398–1404*, 278.
6. *CPL 1398–1404*, 499; *CIPM 1392–99*, nos. 305–7.
7. *CPL 1404–15*, 25; https://www.british-history.ac.uk/vch/cambs/vol2/pp312–314, accessed 12 March 2021.
8. *CPL 1427–47*, 80; *CPL 1471–84*, 237.
9. *PP*, 328.
10. *Fasti Eboracenses*, 382.
11. *CIPM 1235–72*, nos. 317, 365; *Lay Subsidy Roll for the County of Worcester*, ix; *Antiquities of Shropshire*, vol. 1, 186–90.
12. *PROME*: Original Documents, Edward I Parliaments, Roll 11; *CIPM 1235–72*, nos. 551, 706, 881; *CIPM 1272–91*, nos. 178, 212; *CFR 1272–1307*, 76–8, 349, 400; *CIPM 1317–27*, no. 46; *Complete Peerage*, vol. 10, 319–31. Margaret died in 1310 or early 1311; via her son Ralph, she was an ancestor of Edward IV's friend William, Lord Hastings (d. 1483), whose mother was Alice Camoys. William Paynel died on 1 April 1317 leaving his brother John, aged about sixty, as his heir.
13. *CIPM 1307–17*, no. 153.
14. *Wills*, part 2, 186; *LBH*, 35.
15. *CIPM 1352–60*, no. 392.
16. *SPMR*, vol. 2, 32.

17. *Wills*, part 2, 208–9.
18. *CPL 1342–62*, 490; *CPL 1404–15*, 109.
19. *CPL 1198–1304*, 600, 607; *Oxford Dictionary of National Biography*.
20. Karras, 'Sex and the Singlewoman', 141 note 9.
21. *CPL 1417–31*, 289.
22. *CPL 1404–15*, 55; *CPL 1417–31*, 373; *CPL 1471–84*, 106–7.
23. *CPL 1398–1404*, 160, 553.
24. *CCR 1327–30*, 333.
25. Alison Flood, 'Archive shows medieval nun faked her own death to escape convent', *The Guardian*, 11 February 2019; Carol Kuruvilla, 'Medieval nun faked death to pursue 'the way of carnal lust', archives reveal', *Huffington Post*, 12 February 2019; and see https://www.british-history.ac.uk/vch/yorks/vol3/pp129-131#anchorn14, all accessed 22 March 2021.
26. *Liber Albus*, ed. Riley, vol. 1, 396. This same punishment was inflicted on adulterers and adulteresses.
27. *MLL*, 484–6.
28. *EMCR*, 23–4, 184; *Coroner*, 147–8; *CIPM 1405–13*, no. 783; *CIM 1219–1307*, no. 2306.
29. See e.g. *CPL 1362–1404*, 171, 191, 200, 210.
30. *CIM 1308–48*, no. 606.

Chapter 8: Love Language

1. Marvin, 'Medieval Dark Horse', 52.
2. *Medieval English Lyrics*, ed. Davies, 62–3.
3. *Medieval English Lyrics*, 59–61.
4. http://www.luminarium.org/medlit/medlyric/brere.php, accessed 26 April 2021.
5. https://www.bl.uk/collection-items/the-parliament-of-fowls and https://www.bl.uk/learning/timeline/item126579.html, both accessed 22 April 2021.
6. Karras, *Sexuality in Medieval Europe*, 4–5; and see https://quod.lib.umich.edu/m/middle-english-dictionary/dictionary.
7. *CPL 1342–62*, 490.
8. TNA E 101/380/4, fo. 19r.
9. https://anglo-norman.net/entry/a_1, accessed 26 April 2021.

10. *MLLF*, 87; *Coroner*, 39.
11. Middle English Dictionary, https://quod.lib.umich.edu/m/middle-english-dictionary/dictionary, accessed 26 April 2021.
12. https://www.huffpost.com/entry/on-the-origin-of-fuck_b_4784565, accessed 26 April 2021.
13. *CPR 1313–17*, 414 (Fuckere); https://twitter.com/Longshanks1307/status/432856212363694080, accessed 26 April 2021 (Fuckebeggere), and see the Huffington Post article referenced in the note above.
14. Kane, *Impotence and Virginity*, 12–13; https://d.lib.rochester.edu/teams/text/salisbury-trials-and-joys-talk-of-ten-wives-on-their-husbands-ware, accessed 10 May 2021.

Chapter 9: Pregnancy and Childbirth (1)

1. *The Trotula*, ed. Green, 66.
2. Leyser, *Medieval Women*, 96–7.
3. *Trotula*, ed. Green, 66–71, 89–90.
4. Cited in Geaman, 'Struggle to Conceive', 226.
5. *Trotula*, 76–8; *Knowing of Woman's Kind in Childing*, ed. Barratt, 47.
6. Schaus, *Women and Gender*, 167–9; Brundage and Bullough, *Handbook of Medieval Sexuality*, 264.
7. *Trotula*, 78.
8. Riddle, *Eve's Herbs*, 91; Butler, 'Abortion Medieval Style?'. 781–3.
9. *CCR 1302–7*, 231; *CPR 1301–7*, 303; *CPR 1321–24*, 51.
10. For this paragraph, Butler, 'Abortion Medieval Style?', 779–80; Riddle, *Eve's Herbs*, 94–8, 127; Bracton and Fleta quotations in Riddle, 94–5; Richard Bourton's pardon is in *CPR 1327–30*, 113.
11. *SPMR*, vol. 1, 253.
12. TNA SC 8/14/663, SC 8/23/1109.
13. *Coroner*, 20–21, 166–7; *CCR 1339–41*, 354, 359.
14. Trease, 'Spicers and Apothecaries', 37–8, 46. The modern French word for pennyroyal is *pouliot*, and in the document Trease cites, it is called *pewleus*.
15. Carmi Parsons, 'Year of Eleanor of Castile's Birth', 257.
16. *The Trotula*, 77.

Chapter 10: Pregnancy and Childbirth (2)

1. *PROME*, January 1316 parliament.
2. *CIPM 1413–18*, nos. 571–79.
3. *CIPM 1291–1300*, no. 361; *CIPM 1300–07*, no. 213.
4. *Vita Edwardi Secundi*, ed. Denholm-Young, 62.
5. Cited in Jones and Olsan, 'Performative Rituals', 415, 420–1.
6. Maddicott, *Thomas of Lancaster*, 329; Woolgar, *Great Household*, 98; Jones and Olsan, 'Performative Rituals', 424–5.
7. *Trotula*, 73–4, 79–80, 90–1.
8. SAL MS 122, 40, 43.
9. *CIPM 1291–1300*, no. 149; *CIPM 1374–77*, no. 345.
10. *CIPM 1317–27*, no. 435; *CIPM 1352–60*, no. 330; *CIPM 1361–65*, nos. 385, 544; *CIPM 1399–1405*, no. 1180.
11. *CPR 1307–13*, 516, 519.
12. *CIPM 1352–60*, no. 399; *CIPM 1361–65*, no. 379; *CIPM 1365–69*, no. 381; *CIPM 1370–73*, nos. 66–7; *CIPM 1374–77*, no. 343; *CIPM 1399–1405*, no. 999; *CIPM 1442–47*, no. 351.
13. Laynesmith, *Last Medieval Queens*, 115; Delman, 'Gendered Viewing', 184–5.
14. *CIPM 1327–36*, no. 245; *CIPM 1422–27*, no. 829; *CIPM 1437–42*, no. 132.
15. *CIPM 1347–52*, no. 669; *CIPM 1352–60*, no. 535; *CIPM 1399–1405*, nos. 315, 995; *CIPM 1405–13*, no. 900; *CIPM 1427–32*, no. 421; *CIPM 1437–42*, no. 522.
16. *John of Gaunt's Register 1371–75*, nos. 983–84, 1728.
17. *CIPM 1327–36*, no. 253; *CIPM 1352–60*, no. 336; *CIPM 1374–77*, no. 342; *CIPM 1405–13*, no. 996; *CIPM 1437–42*, no. 522; *CIPM 1442–47*, no. 587.
18. Walden Abbey Cartulary, cited in Verity, 'Children of Elizabeth, Countess of Hereford', 7.
19. *CIPM 1272–91*, no. 686; *CIPM 1291–1300*, no. 434; *CIPM 1300–07*, no. 39; *CIPM 1361–65*, no. 543; *CIPM 1365–69*, no. 350; *CIPM 1370–73*, no. 228; *CIPM 1422–27*, nos. 530, 676; *CIPM 1437–42*, no. 130.
20. *CIPM 1413–18*, nos. 654–71.
21. Clark, *Nevills of Middleham*, 74. Cecily's only child Anne Beauchamp was born in February 1444, when Cecily was apparently only 15.

22. See Michèle Schindler's *Lovell Our Dogge: The Life of Viscount Lovell, Closest Friend of Richard III and Failed Regicide* (2019).
23. See https://thewonderoftwins.wordpress.com/2013/07/23/the-significance-of-twins-in-medieval-and-early-modern-europe, accessed 17 April 2021.
24. Mortimer, *Time Traveller*, 207–8.
25. Mortimer, *Time Traveller*, 207.
26. *Trotula*, 92–3, 110.
27. Green and Mooney, 'The Sickness of Women', 461; https://www.reproduction.group.cam.ac.uk/features/sekenesse-of-wymmen, accessed 17 April 2021.
28. Mortimer, *Time Traveller*, 208. See also below, 'Gender Roles and Expectations'.
29. *CIPM 1300–07*, no. 165.
30. *CIPM 1291–1300*, no. 124.
31. *CIPM 1392–99*, no. 955.
32. *CIPM 1365–69*, no. 264.
33. *CIPM 1327–36*, no. 172; *CIPM 1418–22*, no. 874.
34. *CIPM 1422–27*, no. 828; *CIPM 1427–32*, no. 143.
35. *CIPM 1427–32*, no. 673.
36. *CIPM 1413–18*, no. 131.

Chapter 11: Pregnancy and Childbirth (3)

1. *CIPM 1317–27*, no. 188; *CIPM 1327–36*, nos. 124, 251.
2. *CIPM 1422–27*, no. 676.
3. *CIPM 1374–77*, no. 161; *CIPM 1413–18*, no. 272.
4. *CIPM 1361–65*, no. 379; *CIPM 1374–77*, no. 141.
5. *CPL 1342–62*, 460, and see also pp. 489–90 in the same volume.
6. *CPL 1427–47*, 388, 632.
7. *CIPM 1377–84*, no. 883.
8. *CIPM 1352–60*, no. 262.
9. *CIPM 1442–47*, no. 352.
10. *CIPM 1377–84*, no. 159.
11. *CIPM 1307–17*, no. 157; *CIPM 1336–46*, no. 142.
12. *SPMR*, vol. 3, 274; *LBH*, 410; *LBI*, 27.
13. *CIPM 1392–99*, no. 1110; *CIPM 1399–1405*, no. 1140; *CIPM 1405–13*, no. 900; *CIPM 1422–27*, no. 368; *CIPM 1427–32*, no. 136.

14. *CIPM 1374–77*, no. 346; *CIPM 1405–13*, no. 336.
15. *CIPM 1399–1405*, no. 953; *Wills*, part 2, 281.
16. *CIPM 1352–60*, no. 262; *CIPM 1437–42*, no. 131.
17. *CIPM 1399–1405*, no. 314; *CIPM 1418–22*, no. 144; *CIPM 1422–27*, no. 367.
18. *CIPM 1405–13*, nos. 671, 780; *CIPM 1418–22*, no. 758; *CIPM 1427–32*, no. 417; *CIPM 1432–37*, no. 267; *CIPM 1437–42*, nos. 527, 613, 724; *CIPM 1442–47*, nos. 196, 241, etc.
19. *CIPM 1413–18*, no. 263.
20. *CIPM 1413–18*, no. 130; *MLL*, 462.
21. *CIPM 1327–36*, nos. 94, 481; *CIPM 1347–52*, no. 244; *CIPM 1352–60*, no. 336; *CIPM 1422–27*, nos. 531, 664.
22. *CIPM 1317–27*, nos. 192, 336; *CIPM 1327–36*, no. 249; CIPM 1347–52, no. 63; *CIPM 1405–13*, no. 780.
23. *CIPM 1291–1300*, no. 427; *CIPM 1307–17*, no. 151; *CIPM 1352–60*, no. 262; *CIPM 1361–65*, no. 384.
24. *CIPM 1352–60*, no. 334; *CIPM 1399–1405*, no. 998; *CIPM 1437–42*, no. 298; *CIPM 1442–47*, no. 147.
25. *CIPM 1374–77*, no. 300; *CIPM 1437–42*, no. 613; *CIPM 1442–47*, nos. 196, 241.
26. *CIPM 1418–22*, no. 149.
27. *CIPM 1347–52*, no. 124.
28. *CIPM 1370–73*, no. 294.
29. *CIPM 1384–92*, no. 342.
30. *Wills*, part 1, 57, 128, 614; *LBH*, 424; *LBL*, 151.
31. *CPL 1342–62*, 584.
32. *CIPM 1291–1300*, nos. 135, 434; *CIPM 1300–07*, no. 433; *CIPM 1347–52*, no. 122; *CIPM 1361–65*, nos. 381, 542.
33. *CPR 1313–17*, 382; *CIPM 1327–36*, no. 240; *CIPM 1347–52*, nos. 183, 590; *CIPM 1384–92*, nos. 77, 947.
34. *CIPM 1327–36*, no. 395; *CIPM 1352–60*, no. 195; Underhill, *For Her Good Estate*, 95.
35. *CIPM 1352–60*, no. 564; *CIPM 1361–65*, nos. 516, 545; *CCR 1360–64*, 455. Joan was the youngest and only surviving secular child of Alice of Norfolk, beaten to death by her husband Edward Montacute in 1351.
36. *CIPM 1317–27*, no. 333; *CPR 1321–24*, 191, 215–16; *CCR 1318–23*, 591; *CPR 1348–50*, 371; *CIPM 1327–36*, no. 493; *CIPM 1361–65*, no. 614.

37. *CPL 1342–62*, 164, 176, 188; *PP*, 75, 81, 99.
38. *CIPM 1272–91*, no. 743; *CIPM 1291–1300*, no. 623.
39. *CIPM 1317–27*, no. 62; *CIPM 1327–36*, nos. 540, 709; *CIPM 1352–60*, no. 335; *CIPM 1361–65*, no. 548; *CCR 1346–49*, 132.
40. *CIPM 1307–17*, no. 157; *CIPM 1317–27*, no. 754.

Chapter 12: Illegitimacy

1. *CPL 1198–1304*, 247; *CPL 1305–41*, 131, 539; *CPL 1342–62*, 65–7, 72; there are countless other examples.
2. *CPR 1317–21*, 142; *CPR 1338–40*, 132; *CPR 1446–52*, 533.
3. Pollock and Maitland, *History of English Law*, vol. 2, 398.
4. *CPL 1305–41*, 523, 526–7; *PP*, 106, 262.
5. *Oxford Dictionary of National Biography*, and see https://quod.lib.umich.edu/c/cme/Paston/1:8.4?rgn=div2;view=fulltext, accessed 23 March 2021; *he xuld kyt of here nose to makyn here to be know wat sche is, and yf here chyld come in hesse presence he seyd he wyld kyllyn.*
6. *CPR 1313–17*, 401, 434, 528–9; *CPR 1345–48*, 221; TNA SC 8/87/4348; *Testamenta Eboracensia*, vol. 1, 41–5; *CPL 1342–62*, 116, 169, 173; *PP*, 46.
7. *PP*, 491; *CPL 1362–1404*, 175.
8. *CPR 1396–99*, 314; *Testamenta Vetusta*, vol. 1, 85.
9. See my post http://edwardthesecond.blogspot.com/2021/02/laurence-hastings-earl-of-pembroke-d.html.
10. *Coroner*, 130; *CPR 1338–40*, 423; *LBD*, 265.
11. TNA SC 8/50/2489; *CIPM 1384–92*, no. 659; Mortimer, *Fears of Henry IV*, 372.
12. *Wills*, part 1, 593.
13. Isabel of Castile herself was born illegitimate, and her mother María de Padilla, a Castilian noblewoman, was her father's long-term mistress. Isabel and her older sisters Beatriz (who died before she married) and Constanza were legitimised in 1362 after the death of their father's imprisoned French wife Blanche de Bourbon.
14. *PROME*, January 1431 parliament.
15. TNA PROB 11/1/53; *Oxford Dictionary of National Biography*.
16. Steer, 'For Quicke and Deade', 85–7.
17. *CIPM 1291–1300*, no. 213; *Complete Peerage*, vol. 12A, 739.

18. Prestwich, 'An Everyday Story', 151–62; Wells-Furby, *Aristocratic Marriage, Adultery and Divorce*.
19. Prestwich, 'Everyday Story', 153; *CIPM 1327–36*, no. 50.
20. *Calendar of Chancery Warrants 1244–1326*, 199; *CCR 1302–7*, 126; *CPR 1307–13*, 548–9; *CCR 1313–18*, 289; *CPR 1313–17*, 261; *CPR 1340–43*, 398–9; *CIPM 1317–27*, no. 539; *Fasti Eboracenses*, 377; Prestwich, 'Everyday Story', 153–6.
21. *Fasti Eboracenses*, 338.
22. *CIPM 1307–17*, no. 151.
23. *CIPM 1361–65*, no. 268; *CPR 1361–64*, 238–9.
24. *CIPM 1365–69*, no. 156.
25. *Wills*, part 1, 342; *CIPM 1327–36*, no. 223; *LBE*, 239, 250; *LBF*, 75; *SPMR*, 168; *CPR 1324–27*, 1; *CFR 1327–37*, 119; *CIPM 1327–36*, no. 223; *Feet of Fines for London and Middlesex*, vol. 1, Edward II, no. 333.
26. *CIPM 1374–77*, no. 214; *CIPM 1384–92*, nos. 866, 941–2; *CIPM 1392–99*, no. 1114.
27. *CCR 1330–33*, 518–19; *CPR 1343–45*, 311–14; TNA SC 8/118/5891; *Calendar of Documents Relating to Scotland* 1307–57, no. 713.
28. *CCR 1318–23*, 321–2; *CIPM 1307–17*, no. 531; *CIPM 1317–27*, no. 163; *CIPM 1377–84*, nos. 853–8.
29. *Wills*, part 1, 354–5, 689; *CCR 1354–60*, 43; *CCR 1360–64*, 525; *LBE*, 250, 256; *LBH*, 387.
30. *Wills*, part 1, 637–8; *LBI*, 40, 77; *CIPM 1418–22*, no. 806.

Chapter 13: Prostitution

1. Karras, 'Sex and the Singlewoman', 134–5; Karras, *Common Women*, 48 ('constraints' quotation).
2. Karras, *Common Women*, 6–7, 48–9.
3. *London Eyre of 1276*, nos. 119, 134, 181.
4. *LBA*, 218; *EMCR*, 14; *LBB*, 7.
5. *MLL*, 89; *LBD*, 277.
6. *Coroner*, 86, 208–9.
7. *EMCR*, 211, 218–19.
8. *SPMR*, vol. 1, 124–6, 212–13; *SPMR*, vol. 2, 7.
9. *SPMR*, vol. 1, 167, 173, 188.
10. *SPMR*, vol. 2, 151.

11. *MLL*, 484–6.
12. Karras, *Common Women*, 61.
13. Summerson, 'Peacekeepers and Lawbreakers', 107.
14. *Wills*, part 2, 528, and see *MLL*, 20, 267, 458, 488, 535.
15. *LBD*, 242.
16. *La peyne contre putours, baudes, prestres et advoutours; Liber Albus*, vol. 1, 457–60.
17. *LBH*, 372, 402; *MLL*, 534–5.
18. *MLL*, 647–50.
19. Tout, *Place of the Reign*, 280.

Chapter 14: Ravishment and Abduction

1. *Statutes*, vol. 1, 29.
2. Parsons, 'Mothers, Daughters, Marriage', 63–78.
3. *Chronicle of Lanercost*, ed. Maxwell, 85, states that Eleanor was born on the feast of St Andrew, i.e. 30 November, but does not give the year. Her parents married around June 1219 and her older sister Marguerite, Queen of France, was probably born in the spring of 1221.
4. *CPL 1427–47*, 249.
5. *Statutes*, vol. 1, 29.
6. *CPR 1327–30*, 352.
7. *CPR 1317–21*, 278; *CCR 1318–23*, 150–51; TNA SC 8/259/12929; *CIPM 1307–17*, no. 212; *CIPM 1336–46*, no. 27. I have been unable to discover how long John Berenger was imprisoned; he died in 1339, having married and fathered two children, and Elizabeth Percy was still alive in 1351.
8. Tanqueray, 'Conspiracy of Thomas Dunheved', 119–24.
9. Dunn, *Stolen Women*, 2.
10. McSheffrey and Pope, 'Ravishment, Legal Narratives', 818; Dunn, 'Ravishment', 67; Donahue, *Law, Marriage and Society*, 171.
11. *Statutes*, vol. 1, 29, 87: 'if a man ravishes a woman, married, maid or other, where she did not consent, neither before or after, he shall have judgement of life and of member'.
12. *CPR 1321–24*, 139.
13. Cited in Brownmiller, *Against Our Will*, 28.
14. *CPR 1348–50*, 464; *CPR 1350–54*, 358; TNA SC 8/190/9461, SC 8/179/8926, SC 8/181/9042, SC 8/185/9212.

15. *CPR 1348–50*, 566–7; *CPR 1350–54*, 235; *CPR 1361–64*, 43.
16. See for example *CPR 1396–99*, 282; *CPR 1405–8*, 5; *CPR 1408–13*, 42–3, 160, 171, 286.
17. TNA SC 8/146/7252; SC 8/147/7347; *CPR 1381–85*, 197, 236.
18. See Dunn, *Stolen Women*, 48, 83–4, 100–1.
19. *Statutes*, vol. 2, 27; the 'withdrew' quotation is from Kissane, 'Unnatural in Body', 90–1.
20. The Swynnertons' misdeeds appear in my *Living in Medieval England: The Turbulent Year of 1326*, 96, and see 'Plea Rolls for Staffordshire' available on British History Online.
21. 'Plea Rolls for Staffordshire'; *CPR 1307–13*, 228–9, 307.
22. *CPR 1317–21*, 485.
23. TNA SC 8/343/16152.
24. *CPR 1381–85*, 453–4.
25. *CPR 1396–99*, 422; TNA SC 8/252/12568.
26. *CPR 1348–50*, 450.
27. *SPMR*, vol. 2, 5, 23.
28. *CPR 1441–46*, 291, 336.
29. *CPR 1338–40*, 92; *CPR 1350–54*, 121.
30. Kissane, 'Unnatural in Body', 90; see also Karras, *Sexuality in Medieval Europe*, 8.
31. Kissane, 89–90.
32. Dunn, *Stolen Women*, 58, 60, 71.
33. TNA SC 8/87/4307.
34. *CPR 1345–48*, 153; Verity, 'Love Matches', 100, for the Hales family tree.
35. Summerson, 'Peacekeepers and Lawbreakers', 120.
36. *LBL*, 103.

Chapter 15: Incest and Consanguinity

1. A History of the County of York, vol. 3, 163–5, available at https://www.british-history.ac.uk/vch/yorks/vol3/pp163-165, accessed 18 April 2021.
2. *Register of William Melton*, vol. 6, ed. Robinson and Hill, no. 329.
3. https://www.british-history.ac.uk/vch/yorks/vol3/pp182-184, accessed 12 April 2021.
4. *CPL 1342–62*, 167, 173.

5. *CPL 1362–1404*, 441; *CPL 1417–31*, 211.
6. *CPL 1398–1404*, 377.
7. *CPL 1362–1404*, 578.
8. *CPL 1447–55*, 233.
9. *CPL 1342–62*, 116, 169, 173. He had previously tried to have his marriage annulled in 1316 on the grounds that firstly, he was underage when it took place and was 'obliged ... through fear' to marry Jeanne, and secondly, because he was pre-contracted to Maud Nerford: *Fasti Eboracenses*, 384.
10. *CPL 1427–47*, 626.
11. *CPL 1427–47*, 579–80, 635.
12. *Fasti Eboracenses*, 383, 417.
13. *CPL 1198–1304*, 13.
14. *CPL 1471–84*, 835–6.
15. *CPL 1398–1404*, 98–9.
16. *Fasti Eboracenses*, 377; *Registrum Palatinum Dunelmense*, 299, 411, 429, 432, 437, 484.
17. *CPR 1345–48*, 125, 153; TNA SC 8/227/11301. Alice Hales' great-aunt, also Alice Hales, married Edward II's half-brother Thomas of Brotherton in *c.* 1321 and was the mother of Margaret (d. 1399) and Alice (d. 1351) of Norfolk.
18. Verity, 'Love Matches', 100.

Chapter 16: Same-Sex Relationships

1. Karras, *Sexuality in Medieval Europe*, 9.
2. Karras, *Sexuality in Medieval Europe*, 9; Brundage and Bullough, *Handbook of Medieval Sexuality*, 156–7.
3. *Rotuli Parliamentorum*, vol. 2, 332, 350; *PROME*, April 1376 parliament; Cook, ed, *Gay History of Britain*, 23; Ashdown-Hill, *Private Life of Edward IV*, 66–7.
4. Prestwich, 'Court of Edward II', 71.
5. Phillips, *Edward II*, 98.
6. *True Chronicles of Jean le Bel*, trans. Bryant, 31. Despenser's alleged emasculation was not part of the sentence read out at his trial: Holmes, 'Judgement on the Younger Despenser', 261–7.
7. Westerhof, *Death and the Noble Body*, 126–7.
8. Karras, *Sexuality in Medieval Europe*, 148–9.

9. Ashdown-Hill, *Private Life of Edward IV*, 69–77.
10. *The Brut*, ed. Brie, 216–17.
11. *Foedera 1327–44*, 765.
12. Cited in Johnstone, *Edward of Carnarvon*, 42; *Vita Edwardi Secundi*, ed. Denholm-Young, 15.
13. *Flores Historiarum*, 229, and see my *Edward II's Nieces, the Clare Sisters: Powerful Pawns of the Crown* (2020), 108–10, 117–18, 123–4, 131–3.
14. *Historia Anglicana*, vol. 2, ed. Riley, 148; *Oxford Dictionary of National Biography*; *Reign of Richard II*, ed. McHardy, 95–6.

Chapter 17: Gender Roles and Expectations

1. Karras and Boyd, 'Ut Cum Muliere', 99–101; Karras and Linkinen, 'John/Eleanor Rykener Revisited', 112; Bennett and McSheffrey, 'Early, Erotic and Alien', 2–3; Bershady, 'Sexual Deviancy and Deviant Sexuality', 12–13; and see also https://sourcebooks.fordham.edu/source/1395rykener.asp and https://www.publicmedievalist.com/transgender-middle-ages/, both accessed 15 April 2021.
2. See Bennett and McSheffrey, 'Early, Erotic and Alien', for further information about all these women.
3. *LBK*, 94.
4. Karras, *Sexuality in Medieval Europe*, 6.
5. *CPL 1362–1404*, 388–9.
6. *CIPM 1365–69*, no. 87; *CIPM 1442–47*, no. 143; *Prologe of the Wyves Tale of Bathe*, lines 719–807.
7. *Statutes*, vol. 1, 320; *PROME*, January 1352 parliament, *une femme qe tue son baron*.
8. *Complete Peerage*, vol. 9, 85; *CPR 1350–54*, 181, 230; *CCR 1349–54*, 411–12, 459; *CFR 1347–56*, 288, 345; *CPR 1361–64*, 26.
9. *CPR 1301–7*, 280, 344, 427, 472; *CCR 1302–7*, 253. Maud and Thomas's son Richard came of age in 1318 (*CCR 1318–23*, 36), so was about 6 or 7 when his mother killed his father.
10. *CPR 1301–7*, 378, 402, 486; Johnstone, *Letters of Edward, Prince of Wales*, 34, 50–51, 58, 75–6 etc.
11. *Staffordshire Historical Collections*, vol. 6, part 1, ed. G. Wrottesley (1885), 278, 281; *CPR 1350–54*, 175.
12. *CPR 1370–74*, 122; *CPR 1374–77*, 269.

Notes

13. *Coroner*, 87–9, 147–8, 173–4.
14. *SPMR*, vol. 1, 277–8; *LBH*, 10.
15. *LBG*, 175, 216, 297, 306; *MLL*, 368; *SPMR*, vol. 2, 15.
16. *LBI*, 49–50; *LBK*, 124–7.
17. *CPR 1307–13*, 508; *Foedera 1307–27*, 184. Isabella's will does not survive.
18. *SPMR*, vol. 3, 19.
19. *SPMR*, vol. 2, 294.
20. *LBD*, 47.
21. *MLL*, 519–20.
22. *CIPM 1272–91*, no. 37; *CIPM 1370–73*, no. 66..
23. *Wills*, part 1, 189, 266–7, 289–91, 458–9, 474, 495, 557–8, 575, 603, 649–51; *Lincoln Wills*, ed. Foster, 45.
24. Bardsley, 'Missing Women', 274–5.
25. *The Brut*, ed. Brie, part 2, 314; modernised spelling.
26. Hanawalt, *Growing Up in Medieval London*, 56–8, 238 notes 8–11.
27. *CIPM 1336–46*, no. 476; *CIPM 1352–60*, no. 335; *CIPM 1418–22*, no. 758; *CIPM 1437–42*, no. 298.
28. *CPL 1305–41*, 382; *CIPM 1307–17*, no. 67; *CIPM 1327–36*, no. 245; *CIPM 1352–60*, no. 642; *CIPM 1422–27*, no. 530.
29. *CIPM 1422–27*, no. 530.

Bibliography

Primary Sources

The Anonimalle Chronicle 1333–81, ed. V.H. Galbraith (1927; reprinted 1970)
Antiquities of Shropshire, vol. 1, ed. Robert William Eyton (1854)
The Babees' Book: Medieval Manners for the Young, ed. and trans. Edith Rickert and L.J. Naylor (2000)
The Book of Chivalry of Geoffroi de Charny: Text, Context, and Translation, ed. Richard W. Kaeuper and Elspeth Kennedy (1996)
The Book of Holy Medicines, by Henry of Grosmont, first Duke of Lancaster, ed. and trans. Catherine Batt (2014)
The Brut or the Chronicles of England, parts 1 and 2, ed. F.W.D. Brie (1906–08)
Calendar of Chancery Warrants 1244–1326 (1927)
Calendar of Close Rolls, 47 vols., 1251–1454 (1892–1941)
Calendar of Coroners Rolls of the City of London A.D. 1300–1378, ed. R.R. Sharpe (1913)
Calendar of Documents Relating to Scotland, vol. 3, 1307–57, ed. Joseph Bain (1887)
Calendar of Early Mayor's Court Rolls: 1298–1307, ed. A.H. Thomas (1924)
A Calendar to the Feet of Fines for London and Middlesex, vol. 1, ed. W.J. Hardy and W. Page (1892)
Calendar of Inquisitions Miscellaneous, 3 vols. 1219–1377 (1916–37)
Calendar of Inquisitions Post Mortem, 26 vols., 1235–1447 (1904–2009)
Calendar of Letter-Books of the City of London, 11 vols., 1275–1496, ed. R. R. Sharpe (1899–1912)
Calendar of Papal Registers Relating to Great Britain and Ireland: Papal Letters, 14 vols., 1198–1492, ed. W.H. Bliss, C. Johnson and J.A. Twemlow (1893–1960)

Bibliography

Calendar of Patent Rolls, 44 vols., 1258–1452 (1894–1910)
Calendar of Select Plea and Memoranda Rolls of the City of London, 3 vols., 1323–1412, ed. A.H. Thomas (1926–32)
Calendar of Wills Proved and Enrolled in the Court of Husting, London, parts 1 and 2, 1258–1688, ed. R.R. Sharpe (1889–90)
The Chronicle of Lanercost 1272–1346, ed. Herbert Maxwell (1907)
Excerpta Historica, Or, Illustrations of English History, ed. Samuel Bentley (1831)
Fasti Eboracenses: Lives of the Archbishops of York, ed. W.H. Dixon and J. Raine (1863)
Flores Historiarum, vol. 3, ed. H.R. Luard (1890)
Foedera, Conventiones, Litterae, vol. 2, part 2, 1327–44, ed. Thomas Rymer (1821)
John of Gaunt's Register 1371–75, ed. Sydney Armitage-Smith (1911)
John of Gaunt's Register 1379–83, ed. Robert Somerville and Eleanor C. Lodge (1937)
Kirby's Quest for Somerset, Exchequer Lay Subsidies, ed. F.H. Dickinson (1889)
Knighton's Chronicle 1337–1396, ed. G.H. Martin (1996)
The Knowing of Woman's Kind in Childing, ed. Alexandra Barratt (2001)
Lay Subsidy Roll for the County of Worcester, Circa 1280, ed. J.W. Willis Bund (1893)
Liber Albus: The White Book of the City of London, ed. H.T. Riley (1861)
Life-Records of Chaucer, ed. Walford D. Selby, F.J. Furnivall, Edward A. Bond and R.E.G. Kirk (1900)
Lincoln Wills, vol. 1, 1271–1526, ed. C.W. Foster (1914)
Livre de Seyntz Medicines: The Unpublished Devotional Treatise of Henry of Lancaster, ed. E.J. Arnould (1940)
The London Eyre of 1276, ed. Martin Weinbaum (1976)
London Possessory Assizes: A Calendar, ed. Helena M. Chew (1965)
Manuale et Processionale ad Usum Insignis Ecclesiae Eboracensis, ed. William George Henderson (1875)
Medieval English Lyrics: A Critical Anthology, ed. Reginald Thorne Davies (1964)
Memorials of London and London Life in the 13th, 14th and 15th Centuries, ed. H.T. Riley (1868)
National Archives records, especially SC 8 (ancient petitions)

The Parliament Rolls of Medieval England, ed. P. Brand, A. Curry, C. Given-Wilson, R. Horrox, G. Martin, M. Ormrod and S. Phillips (2005)

Petitions to the Pope 1342–1419, ed. W.H. Bliss (1896)

The Register of William Melton, Archbishop of York, 1317–1340, vol. 6, ed. David Robinson and Rosalind M.T. Hill (1977)

Registrum Palatinum Dunelmense: The Register of Richard de Kellawe, Lord Palatine and Bishop of Durham, 1311–1316, vol. 1, ed. T.D. Hardy (1873)

The Reign of Richard II From Minority to Tyranny 1377–97, ed. A.K. McHardy (2012)

Rotuli Parliamentorum, vol. 2, 1327–77 (1769)

Royal and Historical Letters During the Reign of Henry the Fourth, vol. 2, ed. F.C. Hingeston (1860)

Society of Antiquaries of London, Manuscript 122

The Statutes of the Realm, vols. 1 and 2, 1103–1509 (1810–16)

Testamenta Eboracensia, Or, Wills Registered at York, part 1, ed. James Raine (1836)

Testamenta Vetusta: Being Illustrations From Wills, vol. 1, ed. Nicholas Harris Nicolas (1826)

Thomae Walsingham, Quondam Monachi S. Albani, Historia Anglicana, vol. 2, ed. H.T. Riley (1864)

The Trotula: An English Translation of the Medieval Compendium of Women's Medicine, ed. and trans. Monica H. Green (2002)

The True Chronicles of Jean le Bel 1290–1360, trans. Nigel Bryant (2011)

Vita Edwardi Secundi Monachi Cuiusdam Malmesberiensis, ed. N. Denholm-Young (1957)

Secondary Sources

Anglo-Norman Dictionary online, https://anglo-norman.net/entry/a_1

Archibald, Elizabeth, *Incest and the Medieval Imagination* (2001)

Ashdown-Hill, John, *The Private Life of Edward IV* (2017)

Baldwin, David, *Elizabeth Woodville, Mother of the Princes in the Tower* (2002)

Bardsley, Sandy, 'Missing Women: Sex Rations in England 1000–1500', *Journal of British Studies*, 53 (2014), 273–309

Bibliography

Bellamy, John G., *Criminal Law and Society in Late Medieval and Tudor England* (1984)

Bennett, Judith M., and Shannon McSheffrey, 'Early, Erotic and Alien: Women Dressed as Men in Late Medieval London', *History Workshop Journal*, 77 (2014), 1–25

Bershady, Isaac, 'Sexual Deviancy and Deviant Sexuality in Medieval England', *Primary Source*, 5 (2014), 12–18

Bigelow, Melville M., 'The Bohun Wills, II', *The American Historical Review*, 1 (1896), 631–49

Boyd, David Lorenzo, and Ruth Mazo Karras, 'The Interrogation of a Male Transvestite Prostitute in Fourteenth-Century London', *GLQ: A Journal of Lesbian and Gay Studies*, 1 (1995), 459–65

Brownmiller, Susan, *Against Our Will: Men, Women and Rape* (1975)

Brozyna, Martha A., ed., *Gender and Sexuality in the Middle Ages: A Medieval Source Documents Reader* (2005)

Brundage, James A., *Law, Sex and Christian Society in Medieval Europe* (2009)

Brundage, James, and Vern L. Bullough, *Handbook of Medieval Sexuality* (2013)

Bullough, Vern L., 'Transvestites in the Middle Ages', *American Journal of Sociology*, 79 (1974), 1381–94

Butler, Sara M., 'Abortion Medieval Style? Assaults on Pregnant Women in Later Medieval England', *Women's Studies*, 40 (2011), 778–99

Butler, Sara, *The Language of Abuse: Marital Violence in Later Medieval England* (2007)

Butler, Sara, 'Runaway Wives: Husband Desertion in Medieval England', *Journal of Social History*, 40 (2006), 337–59

Cadden, Joan, *Meanings of Sex Difference in the Middle Ages: Medicine, Science, and Culture* (1993)

Clark, K.L., *The Nevills of Middleham: England's Most Powerful Family in the Wars of the Roses* (2016)

Cook, Matt, ed., *A Gay History of Britain: Love and Sex Between Men Since the Middle Ages* (2007)

Dale, Lauren, '*Delictum vel Peccatum?*: An Examination of Legal Cases: Prosecuting Abortion and Infanticide in Medieval England', Master of Research thesis, Keele University (2017)

Delman, Rachel M., 'Gendered Viewing, Childbirth and Female Authority in the Residence of Alice Chaucer, Duchess of Suffolk, in Ewelme, Oxfordshire', *Journal of Medieval History*, 45 (2019), 181–203

Donahue, Charles Jr., *Law, Marriage and Society in the Later Middle Ages* (2008)

Dunn, Caroline, 'Prosecuting Ravishment in Thirteenth-Century England', *Thirteenth Century England XIII*, ed. Janet Burton, Frédérique Lachaud, Phillipp Schofield, Karen Stöber and Björn Weiler (2009), 67–81

Dunn, Caroline, *Stolen Women in Medieval England: Rape, Abduction and Adultery, 1100–1500* (2013)

Geaman, Kristen L., 'A Personal Letter Written by Anne of Bohemia', *English Historical Review*, 128 (2013), 1086–94

Geaman, Kristen L., 'Anne of Bohemia and Her Struggle to Conceive', *Social History of Medicine*, 29 (2016), 224–44

Gibbs, Vicary, ed., *The Complete Peerage*, 14 vols. (1910–40)

Green, Monica H., and Linne R. Mooney, 'The Sickness of Women', *Sex, Aging, and Death in a Medieval Compendium*, ed. M. Teresa Tavormina (2006), 456–568

Hanawalt, Barbara A., *Growing Up in Medieval London* (1993)

Harper, April, and Caroline Proctor, eds., *Medieval Sexuality: A Casebook* (2010)

Holmes, G.A., 'The Judgement on the Younger Despenser, 1326', *English Historical Review*, 70 (1955), 261–7

Huffman, Elizabeth A., 'Marital Incest During the Late Middle Ages in England and Scotland', MA thesis, Iowa State University (1993)

Johnstone, Hilda, *Edward of Carnarvon 1284–1307* (1946)

Johnstone, Hilda, *Letters of Edward, Prince of Wales, 1304–5* (1931)

Johnstone, Hilda, 'The Wardrobe and Household of Henry, Son of Edward I', *Bulletin of the John Rylands Library*, 7 (1920), 384–420

Jones, Peter Murray, and Lea T. Olsan, 'Performative Rituals for Conception and Childbirth in England, 900–1500', *Bulletin of the History of Medicine*, 89 (2015), 406–33

Joseph, Lisa, 'Dynastic Marriage in England, Castile and Aragon, 11th to 16th Centuries', MPhil thesis, University of Adelaide (2015)

Kane, Christina Bronach, *Impotence and Virginity in the Late Medieval Ecclesiastical Court of York* (2008)

Karras, Ruth Mazo, *Common Women: Prostitution and Sexuality in Medieval England* (1996)

Karras, Ruth Mazo, and Tom Linkinen, 'John/Eleanor Rykener Revisited', *Founding Feminisms in Medieval Studies: Essays in Honour of E. Jane Burns*, ed. Laine E. Doggett and Daniel O'Sullivan (2016), 111–21

Karras, Ruth Mazo, *Sexuality in Medieval Europe: Doing Unto Others*, third edition (2017)

Karras, Ruth Mazo, 'Sex and the Singlewoman', *Singlewomen in the European Past 1250–1800*, ed. Judith M. Bennett and Amy M. Froide (1999, reprinted 2013), 127–45

Karras, Ruth Mazo, and David Lorenzo Boyd, 'Ut Cum Muliere: A Male Transvestite Prostitute in Fourteenth-Century London', *Premodern Sexualities*, ed. Louise Fradenburg and Carla Freccero (1996), 99–116

Kissane, Alan, '"Unnatural in Body and a Villain in Soul": Rape and Sexual Violence towards Girls under the Age of Canonical Consent in Late Medieval England', *Fourteenth Century England X*, ed. Gwilym Dodd (2018), 89–111

Laynesmith, J.L., *The Last Medieval Queens: English Queenship 1445–1503* (2004)

Leland, John L., 'Marrying Without Royal License: A Profitable Pardonable Offence', *Medieval Prosopography*, 29 (2014), 75–102

Leyser, Henrietta, *Medieval Women: A Social History of Women in England 450–1500* (2005)

Maddicott, J.R., *Thomas of Lancaster 1307–1322: A Study in the Reign of Edward II* (1970)

Marvin, Andrew, 'The Medieval Dark Horse: Challenge and Reward in the Middle English Lyric', MA thesis, Southern Connecticut State University (2012)

Masters, Sandra, 'Consanguinitas et Ius Sanguinis: Kinship Calculation and Medieval Marriage', MA thesis, Western Michigan University (1994)

Mathew, Gervase, *The Court of Richard II* (1968)

Matthews, Helen, *The Legitimacy of Bastards: The Place of Illegitimate Children in Later Medieval England* (2019)

McCarthy, Conor, *Marriage in Medieval England: Law, Literature and Practice* (2004)

McSheffrey, Shannon, and Julia Pope, 'Ravishment, Legal Narratives, and Chivalric Culture in Fifteenth-Century England', *Journal of British Studies*, 48 (2009), 818–36

Middle English Dictionary online, https://quod.lib.umich.edu/m/middle-english-dictionary/dictionary

Morris, Marc, *The Bigod Earls of Norfolk* (2005)

Mortimer, Ian, *The Fears of Henry IV: The Life of England's Self-Made King* (2007)

Mortimer, Ian, *The Time Traveller's Guide to Medieval England: A Handbook for Visitors to the Fourteenth Century* (2008)

Müller, Wolfgang P., *The Criminalization of Abortion in the West: Its Origins in Medieval Law* (2012)

Myers, Alec Reginald, *The Household of Edward IV: The Black Book and the Ordinance of 1478* (1959)

Niebrzydowski, Sue, *Bonoure and Buxum: A Study of Wives in Late Medieval English Literature* (2006)

Ormrod, W.M., 'Edward III and his Family', *Journal of British Studies*, 26 (1987), 398–422

Parsons, John Carmi, 'Mothers, Daughters, Marriage, Power: Some Plantagenet Evidence, 1150–1500', *Medieval Queenship*, ed. John Carmi Parsons (1998), 63–78

Parsons, John Carmi, 'The Year of Eleanor of Castile's Birth and Her Children by Edward I', *Mediaeval Studies*, 46 (1984), 245–65

Peltzer, Jörg, 'The Marriages of the English Earls in the Thirteenth Century: A Social Perspective', *Thirteenth Century England XIV*, ed. Janet Burton, Philipp Schofield and Björn Weiler (2011), 61–85

Phillips, Seymour, *Edward II* (2010)

Pollock, F., and F.W. Maitland, *The History of English Law*, vol. 2 (second edition, 1898)

Prestwich, Michael, 'The Court of Edward II', *The Reign of Edward II: New Perspectives*, ed. Gwilym Dodd and Anthony Musson (2006), 61–75

Prestwich, Michael, 'An Everyday Story of Knightly Folk', *Thirteenth Century England IX*, ed. Michael Prestwich, Richard Britnell and Robin Frame (2003), 151–62

Prestwich, Michael, 'Royal Patronage Under Edward I', *Thirteenth Century England I*, ed. P.R. Coss and S.D. Lloyd (1986), 41–52

Rees, Willam, *Caerphilly Castle and its Place in the Annals of Glamorgan* (new edition, 1974)

Rhodes, Walter E., 'The Inventory of the Jewels and Wardrobe of Queen Isabella, 1307–8', *English Historical Review*, 12 (1897), 518–21

Bibliography

Riddle, John M., *Eve's Herbs: A History of Contraception and Abortion in the West* (1997)

Salisbury, Joyce E., ed., *Medieval Sexuality: A Research Guide* (1990)

Santos Silva, Manuela, 'The Portuguese Household of an English Queen: Sources, Purposes, Social Meaning', *Royal and Elite Households in Medieval and Early Modern Europe, More Than Just a Castle*, ed. Theresa Earenfight (2018), 271–87

Schaus, Margaret, *Women and Gender in Medieval Europe: An Encyclopedia* (2006)

Smyth, John, *The Lives of the Berkeleys*, vol. 2 (1883; written before 1640)

Some Notes on Medieval English Genealogy: http://www.medievalgenealogy.org.uk/index.html

Sponsler, Claire, 'The King's Boyfriend', *Queering the Middle Ages*, ed. Glenn Burger and Steven F. Kruger (2001), 143–67

Steer, Christian, '"For Quicke and Deade Memory Masses": Merchant Piety in Late Medieval London', *Medieval Merchants and Money: Essays in Honour of James L. Bolton*, ed. Martin Allen and Matthew Davies (2016), 71–89

Sturcken, H.T., 'The Unconsummated Marriage of Jaime of Aragon and Leonor of Castile (October 1319)', *Journal of Medieval History*, 5 (1979), 185–201

Summerson, Henry, 'Peacekeepers and Lawbreakers in London, 1276–1321', *Thirteenth Century England XII*, ed. Janet Burton, Phillipp Schofield and Björn Weiler (2007), 107–21

Tanqueray, F.J., 'The Conspiracy of Thomas Dunheved, 1327', *English Historical Review*, 31 (1916), 119–24

Tompkins, Laura, 'Mary Percy and John de Southeray: Wardship, Marriage and Divorce in Fourteenth-Century England', *Fourteenth Century England X*, ed. Gwilym Dodd (2018), 133–56

Tout, T.F., *The Place of the Reign of Edward II in English History*, second edition (1936)

Trease, G.E., 'The Spicers and Apothecaries of the Royal Household in the Reigns of Henry III, Edward I and Edward II', *Nottingham Mediaeval Studies*, 3 (1959), 19–52

Underhill, Frances, *For Her Good Estate: The Life of Elizabeth de Burgh* (1999)

Verity, Brad, 'The Children of Elizabeth, Countess of Hereford, Daughter of Edward I of England', *Foundations*, 6 (2006), 3–10

Verity, Brad, 'Love Matches and Contracted Misery: Thomas of Brotherton and his Daughters (Part 1)', *Foundations*, 6 (2006), 91–111

Wade Labarge, Margaret, *Mistress, Maids and Men: Baronial Life in the Thirteenth Century* (1965; reissued 2003)

Wells-Furby, Bridget, *Aristocratic Marriage, Adultery and Divorce in the Fourteenth Century: The Life of Lucy de Thweng* (2019)

Westerhof, Danielle, *Death and the Noble Body in Medieval England* (2008)

Wodderspoon, J., *Memorials of the Ancient Town of Ipswich in the County of Suffolk* (1850)

Woolgar, C.M., *The Great Household in Late Medieval England* (1999)

Woolgar, C.M., *The Senses in Late Medieval England* (2006)

Index

abduction 38-42, 45, 98, 109-16
abortion 69-72
adultery 34, 37, 45, 55-61, 67, 98, 105-6, 119-20
age at marriage 9-14, 24, 42
age of parents 10, 14, 92-4
age of consent 108-10
Anne of Bohemia, queen of England 19, 28, 36, 53-4, 112, 127
annulment of marriages 14, 19, 41-5, 47-8, 57, 96, 98, 119, 126
Arderne, John 74
arousal 47, 49, 50, 67
assault, abuse, and domestic violence 45-6, 70-72, 83, 112-13, 115-16, 120-21, 129-30

banns of marriage 13, 15-16, 115, 119
baptisms 83-7
bathing 1-3, 75
bawds 56, 105-6
Beaufort, Margaret, countess of Richmond 10, 92-3
bigamy 22-3
birth aids and customs 74-5
birthdays 83, 86

Book of Holy Medicines, the 50-51, 66
brothels 62, 103-5, 116

Caesarean birth 80
Camoys, John 37, 59, 60
Camville, Aubrey 16, 17, 42-3
celibacy 90, 117
chastity and chaste marriages 51-4
Charny, Geoffroi de 7, 32, 55
Chaucer, Geoffrey 4-5, 15, 28-9, 42, 51, 65, 66-7, 129
child abuse 115-16, 120-21
clandestine marriages 21-2, 118
Clifford, Maud (d. c. 1283) 39, 42, 144-5
clothes and shoes 4-8, 128-9
common scolds 106, 131
common strumpets 41, 104
conception 49, 51, 68-9, 94, 108-9
concubines 61, 63
conjugal debt 51
consanguinity 57, 117-20
contraception 68-9, 90
courtesy of England 10, 36-7

difficult labour 75, 77, 80, 82
dower 11, 23, 36-7, 48, 60

dowry 35-6, 40, 60, 101
droit de seigneur 18

Elizabeth of Rhuddlan, countess of Hereford 9, 16, 78-9, 81
excommunication 22, 43, 45, 48, 70, 118-20
euphemisms 50, 66
examining pregnant women 73-4
explicit language 47, 65-7

family size 90-91
female merchants 132-3
female sexuality 49-50
fertility/infertility 53, 69
forced marriage 38-42
fornication 57, 61

Gaddesden, John 49-50
gender ratios 134-5
gender roles 128-35
gendered language 65-6, 128, 132-3
Giffard, John 16, 17, 39, 42-3, 144-5
godparents 83-6

hairstyles and hair coverings 5-6, 128-9
herbs 2, 3, 50, 54, 69, 72, 75, 80

illegitimacy 15, 44, 60-63, 89-90, 95-102, 126
impediments to marriage 40-41, 45-7, 83-4
impotence 46-7, 67
incest 51, 117-21
inequality 129-31

infant deaths 81-2
infanticide 135
intercourse 49-51, 53, 65-6, 68-9, 80, 108, 122-3, 126

lechery 50, 122-3
Leeds, Joan of 62
lust 32, 50-51, 61-2, 66, 103, 122-3

Magna Carta 52, 111
male and female seed 49
male sexuality 49, 69, 94, 103, 105, 122, 128
marital separation 48
marriages of commoners 12-13, 18
marriages, noble 11-14, 23-5
marriages, royal 10-11, 13-14, 18-19
married women 56, 92, 95, 104, 132
masturbation 49
menstruation 49, 68
midwives 77-8
miscarriages 70-72
Moring, Elizabeth 62, 105
mortality in childbirth and infancy 80-82, 136

Nerford, Margery 45
non-procreative sex 122-3
Norfolk, Alice of 93, 130, 152

Pastons, the 21, 65, 85
Pearl (poem) 136
penetration 66, 115, 122, 128
Perrers, Alice 44, 58, 91
pica 72
pillory 55-6, 63, 105-6, 131-2

170

Index

pleasure 49-51, 66
poetry 64-5
pregnancy 51, 60, 68-72, 80-82, 92-3, 100, 108, 131
premature labour 70-72
primogeniture 133-4
procreative sex 51, 122
proofs of age 92, 129
prostitution 7-8, 47, 63, 66, 103-7, 111, 128
public immorality 55-6, 63
punishment for abduction 42
punishment for adultery 55-6, 63
punishment for assaulting a pregnant woman 70-72
punishment for incest 117, 120
punishment for prostitution 105-6
punishment for rape 110-13
purification/churching 87-8

rank 28-31
rape 53, 109-15, 120-21
rights to a person's marriage 23-7, 32
Rykener, John/Eleanor 128

same-sex relations 122-27
seclusion before and after birth 75-7
second and third marriages 22-3, 32-4
second statute of Westminster 37, 42, 48, 60, 108-10
Sekenesse of Wymmen, the 80
single men and women 48, 56-7, 103, 124-5
smells 3-4, 6
soap 2

step-children 134
stillbirths 10, 46, 70, 71, 80
Summa Confessorum 47
sumptuary laws 7
Swynford, Katherine 29, 58

teeth 3-4
tenants in chief 23-5, 100, 133
transgender people 128-9
Trotula, the 2, 3, 6, 50, 68, 69, 72, 75, 80
twins 78-80

unchaste ecclesiastics 61-3
uterine suffocation 49-50

Valentine's Day 65
verba de futuro 19-20
verba de presenti 19, 22, 119
vice 123, 128
virginity 14, 51-2, 110-11, 119

washing clothes 3, 6
washing and colouring hair 1, 6
wedding clothes 17-18
wedding customs 16-17
wedding dates 18-19
wedding feasts 19
wedding rings 16
wedding vows 16, 19-20
wet-nurses 88-90
widows/widowers 23-6, 29, 30, 32, 36, 47, 50, 52-4, 59, 82, 84
Wife of Bath, the 15, 51, 66, 129
wine 19, 50, 68-9, 75, 86-7
winter weddings 18-19
Woodville, Elizabeth, queen of England 10, 33, 81